An Introduction to Western Medical Acupuncture

For Elsevier

Content Strategist: Poppy Garraway
Content Development Specialist: Veronika Watkins
Project Manager: Julie Taylor
Designer: Ryan Cook
Illustration Manager: Amy Faith Heyden

An Introduction to Western Medical Acupuncture

ADRIAN WHITE, MA MD BM BCh DipMedAc
Clinical Research Fellow (retired)
Plymouth University Peninsula School of Medicine and Dentistry
Plymouth, UK
(formerly) Editor in Chief, Acupuncture in Medicine

MIKE CUMMINGS, MB ChB DipMedAc
Medical Director
British Medical Acupuncture Society
Royal London Hospital for Integrated Medicine
London, UK

JACQUELINE FILSHIE, MBBS FRCA DipMedAc
Consultant in Anaesthesia and Pain Management
The Royal Marsden NHS Foundation Trust
London, UK

Edinburgh London New York Oxford Philadelphia St Louis Sydney Toronto

ELSEVIER
SAUNDERS

ISBN 978-0-7020-7318-2
e_ISBN 978-0-7020-7511-7

Notices
Knowledge and best practice in this field are constantly changing. As new research and experience broaden our understanding, changes in research methods, professional practices, or medical treatment may become necessary.
Practitioners and researchers must always rely on their own experience and knowledge in evaluating and using any information, methods, compounds or experiments described herein. Because of rapid advances in the medical sciences, in particular, independent verification of diagnoses and drug dosages should be made. To the fullest extent of the law, no responsibility is assumed by Elsevier, authors, editors or contributors for any injury and/or damage to persons or property as a matter of products liability, negligence or otherwise, or from any use or operation of any methods, products, instructions, or ideas contained in the material herein.

Printed in Great Britain
Last digit is the print number: 10 9 8 7 6 5 4 3

CONTENTS

At a challenging moment for healthcare, where robust evidence is needed to introduce any new technique into practice and scepticism about everything 'alternative' is rife, acupuncture is facing a testing time. When put together with the staunchly held beliefs of the traditionalists, a clash between the 'Evidence Base' and the 'Traditional' school is inevitable, making the challenge even more onerous.

Acupuncture is a therapeutic system that developed through observation and clinical experience processes that spawn personal opinions. Charisma, experience, the arrogance of presumed or self-proclaimed authority and clinical application guided its evolution and moulded the principles which all of us who decided to study it were introduced to. What we should not forget though, as W. Edwards Deming once said: "Without data, it's just an opinion."

Acupuncture has evolved in recent years to become a useful and effective tool in the arsenal of the musculoskeletal pain therapist. Frequently, its foundation in Traditional Chinese Medicine (TCM) creates friction with an establishment whose point of reference is the Western Medical model. Nevertheless, as evidence for its physiological and clinical effects becomes available, its acceptance as a valid, biologically plausible method of treatment is increasing. The bio-medical model of clinical reasoning, as proposed in Western medical acupuncture, seems to be the most promising development in the field of acupuncture, or needling-based therapies in general.

In years gone by, the excitement of seeing a new title in the bookshop (I am of an age when bookshops were where we went to get books…) was often quickly replaced by disappointment when one found the 'same old stuff', rehashed, repackaged, and regurgitated with alarming regularity. So, when I was asked to write the foreword for 'Introduction to Western Medical Acupuncture', the cynicism of age and experience made me cast a doubtful eye on its cover.

But one is never too old nor too experienced to be surprised. I certainly was (not too old – surprised!): here is a text that offers a clear, concise, and evidence-based view of acupuncture, both theory and practice.

What this book manages to achieve is to bridge those two worlds and state the obvious: times have changed and the two schools should learn from each other if the practice of acupuncture is to grow and continue to benefit patients in the years to come.

It is obviously written with the busy modern health professional in mind, who already practises or is currently being trained to use acupuncture. Divided into clear sections that follow each other in logical order, it uses an informal but not casual way to communicate its messages. It is accessible and quickly imparts the information it contains. Sections covering scientific aspects of acupuncture are concise, informed, clear, and current, and are presented in an understandable way – by no means an easy feat. But, seeing the list of authors, this is no surprise: experienced researchers, clinicians and educators, with a firm background in Western principles of science and a deep understanding of the practice of acupuncture, they are the ideal folk to grapple with the task at hand.

The sections dealing with the various approaches to needling (myofascial trigger points, traditional Chinese acupuncture) are also very clear, as well as being described and discussed in an impartial way. The presentation of the evidence base for acupuncture as a treatment of various conditions is similarly well researched, objective and detailed. Conveniently divided into sections relating to individual conditions, it can act as a quick reference guide. The sections on the practical aspects of treatment and the treatment manual, along with the quick reference cards that accompany the book, are also useful for the less experienced or the recently trained.

All in all this is a remarkable book. Its structure, language, simplicity in its approach, and comprehensive examination of acupuncture theory and practice should establish it as THE modern manual of Western medical acupuncture.

Panos Barlas

There are numerous textbooks devoted to acupuncture, covering both theoretical and practical aspects of the therapy. The majority of books focus on traditional theory and practice, but this one takes quite a different view. It combines the latest ideas about the neurophysiological mechanisms of acupuncture with a practical approach that is directed largely by those mechanisms. Classical point locations and names are retained because they are useful and well known, but this book lays much greater emphasis on their segmental innervation than on any concepts of meridians.

Western medical acupuncture is used following an orthodox diagnosis and applies scientific principles, taking account of this diagnosis, to formulate a treatment to relieve symptoms. It is just one therapeutic method alongside others and fits perfectly into the wider approach of the whole of Western medicine, which considers both the psychosocial and the physical well-being of the individual.

Thus, Western medicine that includes this form of acupuncture is one example of truly integrated medicine: a traditional therapy has been investigated, reinterpreted within a modern scientific context, and finally incorporated, where appropriate, within modern health care.

This book is a companion to *Medical Acupuncture: a Western Scientific Approach*.

ACKNOWLEDGEMENTS

This book represents the ideas, knowledge and wisdom of many people, and the authors are grateful to everyone with whom they have had conversations or whose articles they have read or lectures they have heard, and who have contributed in some way or other to this work, which tries to make sense of acupuncture in terms of Western science. They are literally too many to list here, and the references at the end of the book give some indication of the number and diversity of researchers who are engaged in the project of understanding acupuncture. We are also grateful for the help, patience and professionalism of Nicola Lally, Poppy Garraway and Veronika Watkins at Elsevier.

Despite the best intentions of all the above, we willingly accept responsibility for any errors or omissions.

Please note: a list of classical meridians and their standard abbreviations appears in Tables 19.6 and 19.7 on page 211. Additional information and other definitions relating to pain can be seen on the IASP Taxonomy website: www.iasp-pain.org/Taxonomy

action potential: A nerve's electrical response to stimulation; for example, by an acupuncture needle. The action potentials travel (or 'propagate') along the nerve fibre to the synapse (see below)

acupuncture point: Traditionally, a precise location where needles may be inserted; in Western medical acupuncture, needling is not limited to traditional acupuncture points

acute/chronic pain: Pain of less than/more than 3 months duration, though some authorities prefer 6 months (see also 'sensory (component of pain)')

affective (component of pain): The emotional aspect of pain, which is troubling or upsetting; 'the pain is awful' (see also 'sensory')

afferent nerve: A nerve that brings information from the periphery towards the central nervous system – sensory nerve (from the Latin for 'bring towards')

allodynia: Pain caused by a stimulus that does not normally provoke pain

analgesia: Analgesia strictly means complete removal of pain, but 'acupuncture analgesia' means pain reduction, often used in conjunction with conventional anaesthesia

associative cortices: Cortical areas that underlie our experience of the world; they are distinguished from 'primary' cortices that are concerned directly with sensory or motor activity

auricular acupuncture: Acupuncture in which needles are inserted into the external ear

autonomic nerves: Nerves responsible for controlling the body's functions that are not within conscious control

central nervous system (CNS): Nervous system situated within spinal column and skull, i.e. spinal cord and brain

channel (meridian): Invisible lines on the surface of the body connecting acupuncture points. No physical structure to explain these channels has been found. In traditional Chinese medicine, channels are believed to be the route for the flow of '*qi*'; also meridian

collateral (fibre): Secondary neuronal fibre projecting to a different target from the principal axon

convergence: The merging of input from several different sources into a single cell or nucleus in the CNS

de qi: Chinese word for needle sensation, literally 'numbness, distension, heaviness and ache'; also tingling and spreading sensation

dermatome: The area of body surface innervated by sensory nerves from a single spinal segment

dorsal horn: The part of the grey matter within the segment of the spinal cord where primary afferent nerves terminate

dry needling: A term sometimes used for acupuncture when needling is performed without a traditional Chinese approach

efferent nerve: A nerve that carries information away from the central nervous system, either motor or autonomic

electroacupuncture: Electrical stimulation applied through needles inserted in the usual way

heterotopic noxious conditioning stimulus (HNCS): Painful stimulation of the periphery that activates widespread descending inhibition of pain. Formerly known as diffuse noxious inhibitory control, DNIC

hyperalgesia: Increased pain from a stimulus that normally provokes pain

laser 'acupuncture': Low-energy laser applied to acupuncture points, without needles

limbic system: Collection of several centres within the brain which are closely involved in various emotional responses

major points: Acupuncture points that seem to have particularly strong generalized regulatory or stimulatory effects

meridian: See 'channel'

modulate : To modify the function of a cell, nucleus or organ in any direction

moxa: Dried leaf of the plant *Artemisia vulgaris* used as a thermal stimulus. It is burnt either directly over the skin or on or close to a needle. This procedure, *moxibustion*, was an integral part of traditional Chinese acupuncture

myelinated: Referring to nerve: covered in myelin sheath which increases speed of transmission

myofascial trigger point: Small area of hyperirritability within a taut band of skeletal muscle that has particular characteristics

myotome: All the muscles innervated from a single spinal segment

NADA technique: Standardized form of auricular acupuncture for drop-in treatment centres for drug addicts, developed by the National Acupuncture Detoxification Association

neuropeptides: Small molecules used by neurons to communicate with each other via surface receptors. Unlike neurotransmitters, they are not taken up again and recycled but broken down in extracellular space. Opioid peptides are neuropeptides that are intimately concerned with the actions of acupuncture. Other examples are CGRP, NGF, noradrenalin, serotonin, oxytocin, cholecystokinin, VIP, substance P.

neuropathic pain: Type of pain caused by damage or disease of the somatosensory nervous system

neuroplasticity: Change to the functioning of nervous system in response to stimulus, especially repeated stimulus

neurotransmitter: Any chemical within the body that stimulates a nerve, and particularly a chemical released by another nerve locally (neurotransmission)

nociceptor: A high-threshold sensory receptor of the peripheral somatosensory nervous system that is capable of transducing and encoding noxious stimuli

nociception: The neural process of sensing a stimulus that could be harmful to the body; it may (or may not) give rise to the perception of pain

opioid peptides: A class of endogenous chemical transmitter within the CNS, whose overall effect is to reduce the perception of pain

pain: An unpleasant sensory and emotional experience associated with actual or potential tissue damage, or described in terms of such damage

periosteal pecking: Stimulation of the periosteum with a needle

percutaneous electrical nerve stimulation: Effectively, the same treatment as electroacupuncture, though not necessarily using acupuncture points

placebo: An intervention that pretends to be a physical or chemical treatment but works entirely psychologically; use of placebo without patient consent is considered unethical

project (verb): Of a nerve: to make synapse with and have influence over (another neuron)
propagate: Correct term to describe the movement of action potentials along a nerve fibre

receptive field: The region (usually skin) from which a peripheral nerve can be excited

qi **('chi'):** A traditional term often translated as 'energy'; originally represented nourishment and defence of the body (i.e. modern-day equivalent is blood supply and immune function)

sclerotome: The area of bone innervated by sensory nerves from a single spinal segment
sensitization: Increased responsiveness of nociceptive neurons to their normal input, and/or recruitment of a response to normally subthreshold inputs. This can be peripheral or central, or commonly both
sensory stimulation: Treatments, including acupuncture, that involve stimulation of the sensory nerves.
sensory (component of pain): The awareness of the pain in terms of site, nature and intensity: 'It hurts here' (see also 'affective' for psychological effect)
sensory stimulus: A physical modality that results in activation of sensory nerves
sham: Pretend, usually in the context of a pretend treatment that is designed as a control procedure in a clinical trial
somatic: To do with the 'soma', which is basically the musculoskeletal parts of the body as distinct from the visceral parts
somatovisceral: The effect the body may have on the internal organs by neural pathways
strong reactor: A patient who has much stronger adverse and beneficial reactions to acupuncture than most people
substantia gelatinosa: Outer part of dorsal horn where afferent nociceptive fibres terminate
superficial needling: Needles enter the skin and superficial fascia but do not penetrate deeper
synapse: The junction between two nerve cells, where the action potential in the first may transfer to the second, propagating the stimulus. The synapse is the crucial site where activity of the nervous system can be modified: local circumstances determine whether the effect of the incoming stimulus may be reduced, blocked or amplified

tender point: A location that causes pain when pressed; may or may not have the specific features of a myofascial trigger point
TENS: Transcutaneous electrical nerve stimulation, a technique of sensory stimulation through surface electrodes. Differs from acupuncture in important ways, especially in not (usually) having sustained or cumulative effects
traditional Chinese acupuncture: An acupuncture approach that embraces various different models of acupuncture that evolved in different parts of China and at different historical periods. Part of traditional Chinese medicine (TCM)

viscerotome: All the organs innervated by the sensory nerves from a single spinal segment
viscerosomatic: The reflex effect that events in the internal organs have on the rest of the body by neural pathways

Western medical acupuncture: An acupuncture approach that interprets acupuncture phenomena according to current understanding of the body's structure and function and integrates acupuncture with Western medicine

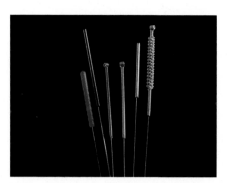

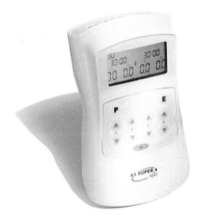

Plate 1 Acupuncture needles showing the development of different types of handles over several years. The old-fashioned, double-wound solid silver was superseded by wound silver, then stainless steel or copper and more recently plastic.

Plate 2 An example of a typical modern electropuncture stimulator, which is used to stimulate needles in Western acupuncture instead of the strong manual stimulation that was used by Chinese acupuncturists.

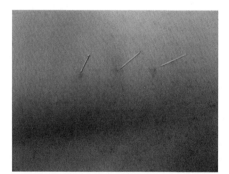

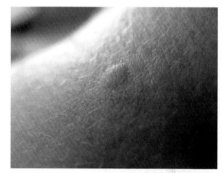

Plate 3 Flares developing in the tissues surrounding a needle, which indicate that the local blood supply is increased through a local nerve reflex.

Plate 4 Close-up view of a weal after removal of the acupuncture needle. The weal is the result of fluid leakage from the small blood vessels – another sign of the local response to acupuncture.

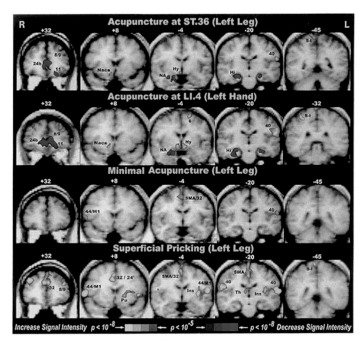

Plate 5 Functional magnetic resonance image of brain activation showing response of various limbic system centres in nine patients given acupuncture at LI4, acupuncture at ST36, minimal acupuncture (superficial needling over an acupuncture point) or superficial pricking elsewhere. Yellow-red colours indicate increased activity of nucleus accumbens (Nacs) and hypothalamus (Hy), as well as areas in sensory cortex. Green-blue colours indicate decreased activity at amygdala (NA) and hippocampus (Hi). Numbers above each image indicate distance in mm from anterior commissure. Numbers in cortical areas of the images correspond to Brodmann areas. *(Reproduced with permission from Wu et al., 1999. Central nervous pathway for acupuncture stimulation: localization of processing with functional MR imaging of the brain – preliminary experience. Radiology 212(1), 133–141.)*

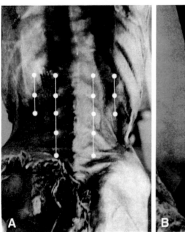
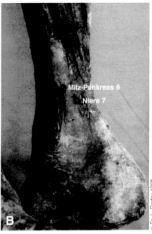

Plate 6 Photographs of the body of Ötzi (the Ice Man) showing (A) tattoos on the back in strikingly similar location to the classical acupuncture points that have been superimposed; and (B) tattoos on the medial aspect of the lower leg in the location of SP6 (Milz-Pankreas 6) and KI7 (Niere 7). *(Reproduced with kind permission of Dr. L. Dorfer.)*

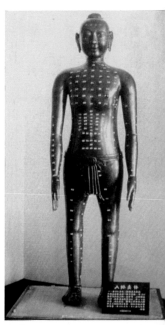

Plate 7 Hollow bronze statue showing acupuncture points. This is a photograph of a reproduction of the original statue cast in 1443 AD during the Ming Dynasty

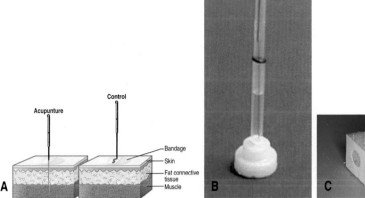

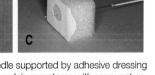

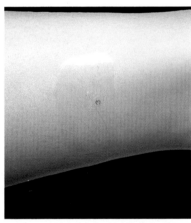

Plate 8 Various forms of placebo device and support: (A) Streitberger needle supported by adhesive dressing *(reproduced with permission from Martin et al., 2006. Improvement in fibromyalgia symptoms with acupuncture: results of a randomized controlled trial. Mayo Clin Proc 81(6), 749–757)*; (B) Park needle supported by guide tube and adhesive flange *(reproduced with kind permission of Dr. Jongbae Park)*; (C) blunt needle with adhesive surgical foam as support. *(Reproduced with kind permission of Dr. Mathias Fink.)*

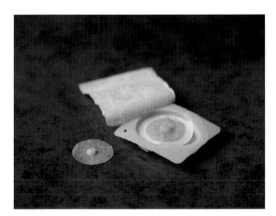

Plate 9 Photograph of an acceptable indwelling needle embedded in plastic with dressing attached, also showing its packaging.

Plate 10 Indwelling acupuncture needle supplied with adhesive plaster.

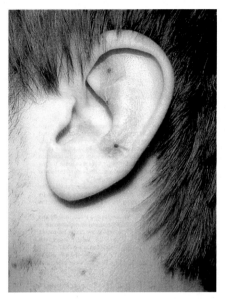

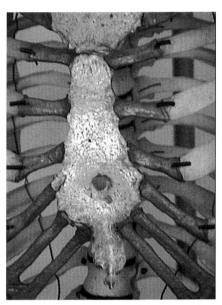

Plate 11 Photograph of Vaccaria seeds used for auricular stimulation.

Plate 12 Photograph of foramen sternale. *(Reproduced with kind permission of Dr. Panos Barlas.)*

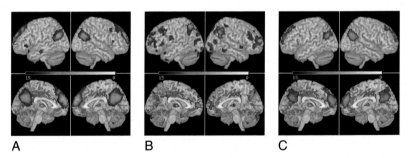

A   B   C

Plate 13 (A) The default mode networks (DMNs) of healthy volunteers during rest, comprised of the inferior parietal lobule, posterior cingulate cortex and medial areas of the inferior, middle and superior frontal gyri, and the precuneus. (B) The DMN connectivities in patients with chronic low back pain (cLBP) before treatment were reduced in the dorsolateral prefrontal cortex, medial prefrontal cortex, anterior cingulate gyrus, and precuneus, as compared with the control group. (C) After treatment the DMNs of the patients with cLBP were almost identical to those of the control group. *(Reproduced with permission from Li, J., et al, 2014. Acupuncture treatment of chronic low back pain reverses an abnormal brain default mode network in correlation with clinical pain relief. Acupuncture in Medicine 32(2), 102–108.)*

Introduction

Treatment with acupuncture is a strange experience. Before lying down on the treatment couch, patients may be asked to roll up their sleeves and take off their socks or stockings – even though they are not complaining of anything wrong with their hands and feet. The acupuncturist will probably prod them in various parts of the body and perhaps measure along the skin with his or her fingers, looking for a particular point to insert some special needles. The insertion itself is not likely to hurt at all – and certainly not like the sharp prick that you might expect – which is just as well, because the acupuncturist will go on inserting more needles, possibly as many as six or eight. The needles go either just into the skin or deeper into the muscle. Each needle is about 1 inch long (Plate 1) and is inserted up to about halfway and then may be twiddled for 30 seconds or so. This produces an odd kind of ache, which is strange because the needles are solid – nothing is being injected and nothing is drawn out. Then the needles just rest there, or sometimes they are attached to a battery-powered stimulator (Plate 2), which causes a gentle tingle. The needles are left for about 10 to 20 minutes before simply being taken out again. The patient then goes home, often feeling relaxed for a few hours, even a bit sleepy. Then he or she may notice that the symptoms feel a bit better – though, just as likely, not after only one treatment. This performance is repeated once a week for a course of six or eight treatments, and in most cases the symptoms gradually disappear.

Patients who ask their acupuncturist what acupuncture is about, or who explore acupuncture on the Internet or in a book, will probably be told about acupuncture's origins in traditional Chinese medicine. They will also be told that the needles work by influencing something called 'qi' energy, which flows round the body in structures called 'meridians'. These unusual concepts (which are not supported by evidence, by the way) seem to match the strangeness of the treatment, and so they tend to be accepted, even sometimes by people who recognize that they are completely foreign to the Western understanding of the way the body works. These explanations even seem to be accepted by some health professionals, which makes it easier for patients to accept them uncritically, thinking: 'The professionals should know, so why question them?'

Readers of this book will discover a different approach: we take this strange therapy that has grown over many centuries, and we try to reinterpret it in modern terms. We use a scientific viewpoint and apply the present-day understanding of how the body works to explain what happens when those needles are inserted and manipulated. Acupuncture works by stimulating sensory nerves, the same ones used by sensations like touch, pressure, stretch and even pain. We hope to show that this medical approach can be used not only to explain what happens during acupuncture, but also as a guide to how to treat various conditions with needles. We hope this style of acupuncture will be more readily accepted in Western medicine and therefore become more widely available to patients.

Let us summarize the position we take in this book:

- Acupuncture is a useful treatment that deserves a place alongside conventional drugs and surgery, and physical and psychological therapies too.
- There is a valid, modern approach to acupuncture that views it as a form of stimulation of nerve and muscle.
- We are not saying that our particular explanations are 'right' and traditional Chinese explanations are 'wrong'.
- We are not saying that science has provided all the answers – there are still plenty of gaps in our knowledge and understanding.
- The scientific approach is the best way to increase knowledge and understanding of acupuncture in the future, because it is self-critical by its very nature.

How can we be sure acupuncture is a valid therapy?

Acupuncture has often been dismissed without giving it much thought. After all, it is a really unfamiliar treatment and quite unlike any other treatment in the whole of medicine or surgery, and the usual explanations given for it are even odder. So we can understand when people think, 'It must be just suggestion'. We have our fair share of scepticism, but our experience with acupuncture convinces us that it is a real and valuable phenomenon. Here are just three lines of reasoning in support of that view:

1. Acupuncture is increasing in popularity, both among patients and among their doctors – some of whom have a reputation for being pretty hard-headed. The opinions of so many thousands of sensible people should not be dismissed too easily. A UK survey of practitioners published in 2009 estimated that about 4 million acupuncture treatments were given each year, a third of which were within the National Health Service (Hopton et al., 2012). Acupuncture is offered to patients in 84% of chronic pain clinics in the National Health Service (Woollam and Jackson, 1998). In these pain clinics, competition for resources is intense and no treatment survives unless it works reasonably frequently. Nearly half of older patients with back pain have tried acupuncture (Greville-Harris et al., 2016). Acupuncture is increasingly used by general practitioners (GPs) themselves, or provided by other members of the primary healthcare team. Acupuncture is one of the most popular complementary therapies. A similar picture emerges from other Western countries such as Australia (Wardle et al., 2013), and acupuncture continues to be offered routinely in many countries in the East, such as China, Korea and Vietnam (Chang et al., 2011; Pham et al., 2013), often in parallel with mainstream Western-style medicine.

2. There is increasing evidence from clinical trials that acupuncture is not just a placebo. There are many difficulties in organizing rigorous clinical trials of acupuncture, and not the least of these is what to use as the 'placebo'– after all, what else looks and feels like a needle, but is not a needle? However, there are now enough trials, and reviews of those trials, to be reasonably confident that acupuncture has real effects. Reviews have shown acupuncture to be better than sham controls in treating different kinds of problems, including high-quality evidence on neck and back pain, osteoarthritis and headaches (Vickers et al., 2012), as well as nausea and vomiting (Lee et al., 2015). There is plenty of evidence of its effectiveness in other conditions, and we summarize these later in the book.

3. Perhaps the most powerful argument in favour of acupuncture is the accumulated clinical experience that comes with watching patients being treated with acupuncture and listening to their comments. The events that happen, both during and after treatment, are so distinctive and so unexpected that patients simply could not make them up. And these events happen

---

Box 1.1 ■ Phenomena that are characteristic of acupuncture treatment

- The needles may produce sensations quite unlike anything else ever experienced.
- Pain relief occurs in three distinct patterns: sometimes immediately on removing the needles; sometimes the morning after treatment; and sometimes gradually accumulating over a course of several treatments.
- Needles in one part of the body treat another part (e.g. patients with migraines benefit from being needled in the foot).
- Patients spontaneously report feelings of improved well-being and deep sleep after treatment.
- Other minor symptoms (not known to the acupuncturist and quite incidental to the main problem being treated) are often improved by acupuncture, such as an irregular menstrual cycle or a mild bowel disorder.
- Mild 'systemic' adverse events may occur after treatment (e.g. drowsiness, aggravation of symptoms, headache or nausea).
- Very occasionally, acupuncture produces a surprisingly strong impact on the nervous system, causing powerful emotional reactions.

---

often enough and are similar enough in completely different patients to suggest that acupuncture needles have some quite definite and biological effects. Some of these events are listed in Box 1.1.

Why not simply accept the traditional explanations for acupuncture?

People tell us that, because the Chinese discovered acupuncture many centuries ago and are still using it, and because their explanations are so natural, beautiful and philosophical, they must be right. The same people tell us that our scientific approach is too limited to do justice to the subtleties of this ancient art. We are not convinced by this and shall explain why here, briefly (and in more detail later in the book).

Acupuncture developed over the course of 2000 years. During this period, theories about the world evolved and changed dramatically as people made new discoveries and achieved a fresh understanding of nature. With each new world view, the phenomena of acupuncture were explained in a different way, according to the new ideas. We are simply continuing this tradition.

Until now, acupuncturists have been careful not to reject the earlier concepts but to add the new explanations on to the old. So, ancient Taoist concepts of yin and yang from naturalism circa 300–400 BC, incorporated during the era of Han Confucianism circa 100 BC, mingle with ideas of disease due to possession by demons, theories of five fundamental universal elements and modern syndromes. There seems to have been a kind of respect for earlier models that made people hang on to the old ideas as some kind of insurance against losing valuable insights.

However, Western science has brought a whole fundamental change to the nature of our knowledge and understanding, and to keep hold of the old ideas while adding the new ones would be the equivalent of asking the reader to accept both that the world is round *and* that it is flat. That is not easy for the modern person.

We regard traditional Chinese acupuncture as a fascinating part of the history of medicine, and we respect the ancient physicians, but their explanations are not meaningful today – at least, not to us. We shall illustrate this with just three examples of fundamental ideas in traditional Chinese acupuncture theory:

1. Traditional Chinese acupuncture involves the basic concept that acupuncture points exist on meridians, and it is through the meridians that the needles achieve their effects. But

nobody has shown any evidence for the physical existence of these meridians, so far. To get round this problem, the meridians are sometimes described as only an abstract concept, but it is difficult to accept how such an abstract concept can have the powerful physiological effects that we see in clinical practice.

2. Traditional Chinese acupuncture can offer an explanation for every individual's symptoms and can offer a diagnosis for every condition in the medical dictionary. However, from what we know about the huge range of diseases that are known to medicine, it seems highly improbable that conditions as different as cancer, rheumatoid arthritis, pneumonia and heart disease can be explained by a single, all-embracing mechanism, let alone that they might all respond to treatment with acupuncture needles.

3. When it comes to the actual treatment with acupuncture, the points are selected on the basis that every acupuncture point has a specific function. For example, a point near the great toe 'clears Liver-Fire'. Even if we can understand the symptoms of 'Liver-Fire' as hot sensations and flushing of the skin, the idea that the underlying cause of these sensations can be corrected by needling a specific point in the foot is not meaningful, according to what we know of the anatomy and physiology of the body. This 'cause-and-effect' relationship seems to be the territory of science, not a traditional belief system, and explanations using the ideas that the needles stimulate nerves and release transmitters in the brain seem to us to be much more appropriate.

Readers will be forgiven for reaching the conclusion that, if they wanted to accept the theory of traditional Chinese acupuncture, they would have to 'suspend their disbelief'. It is time to reconsider acupuncture and its strange phenomena in ways that are credible to Western science.

What this book offers

So this is the heart of our argument: acupuncture works, but not for the reasons usually stated. Acupuncture as a treatment is valid, but the traditional explanations do not apply in the modern world.

The aim of this book is to provide explanations that tie in with current understanding of structure, function and disease – plus a small amount of conjecture. We accept that these explanations are only provisional and will be revised when new discoveries are made, but they provide a sound basis for treatment that is rational in the present circumstances. We believe this approach will make acupuncture accessible to many more patients.

It is not our aim to write a 'cookbook' of treatment recipes, but to help the reader understand the fundamental principles of acupuncture that can then be applied to any situation in which it is appropriate.

The arrangement of the book unfolds our understanding of acupuncture progressively, and to some extent the later chapters assume that the reader understands the topics covered in the previous chapters. We have written the book for practitioners, and however experienced the practitioner may be in other areas of health, we strongly urge everyone to read the information on *safety* carefully: needles can be dangerous, but acupuncture is very safe in the correct hands. We put an emphasis on safety by including one chapter on the evidence and a second chapter on safe practice.

The book lays out the underlying principles in Section 1: principles of acupuncture itself, of pain and the nervous system, and of clinical practice of acupuncture. Section 2 describes the effects of acupuncture and is organized to reflect *treatment approaches* – that is, where to place the needle and how to stimulate it. There are three targets for treatment:

- local – tissue changes and local reflexes
- segmental – based on the spinal reflexes
- general – changes to various centres in the brain, affecting the whole body

Within each of these targets, the treatment approach can be modified to achieve different effects. Local needling can aim to improve blood supply or to inactivate myofascial trigger points; segmental needling might aim to reduce pain or to modulate the autonomic nervous system; and general effects can include descending pain inhibition or wider, hormonal and behavioural effects. Naturally, needles might achieve more than one effect simultaneously.

Section 3 summarizes the evidence of safety and effectiveness, and Section 4 covers how the patient and the practitioner should be prepared for practice. Finally, Section 5 gives some practical guidelines for treating different conditions and provides reference charts for referral patterns of myofascial trigger points, as well as locations of the most important of the classical points.

Who should use this book?

This book is intended for people who want to learn how to use acupuncture in their treatments. It must be seen as a supplement to practical 'hands-on' training courses for healthcare practitioners and not as a substitute. Learning any practical therapy such as acupuncture must involve some observation and apprenticeship.

In line with the principle of 'first do no harm', we urge readers to always make sure that a patient who is considering acupuncture has had a conventional medical consultation. Acupuncture might reduce symptoms temporarily and therefore critically delay the diagnosis or treatment. For example, acupuncture might alleviate an organ dysfunction, but if that dysfunction is caused by infection, inflammation, cancer, ischaemia, degeneration or a mechanical problem such as intestinal obstruction, then the improvement will be short-lived and precious time will have been lost.

Many terms in acupuncture – as well as in anatomy and physiology – that are used throughout the book may be new to the reader. Instead of defining such terms each time they appear, we provide a glossary at the start.

Finally, a note of caution on the use of literature references in this book. It is not feasible to provide comprehensive scientific citation to support every factual statement we make, or the reference list would be longer than the text. We have tried to cite references to support all crucial steps in the arguments, and we have also tried to include all the major references that we believe will be useful to any reader who wishes to expand his or her knowledge on particular subjects. Readers wanting a more rigorous academic approach should consult the companion book, listed in Further Reading.

Further reading

Filshie, J., White, A., Cummings, M. (Eds.), 2016. Medical acupuncture: a Western scientific approach. Elsevier, Edinburgh.
    This multi-author textbook, a companion to the Introduction to Western Medical Acupuncture, provides detailed information, written by experts, on the mechanisms of acupuncture and its usage and effectiveness in a wide range of conditions.

Principles

An overview of Western medical acupuncture

Introduction

To a casual observer, Western medical acupuncture looks very similar to traditional Chinese acupuncture. Needles are inserted in various places in the body, often including the hands and feet. The needles are agitated by hand and sometimes stimulated by electrical impulses, and they are taken out again after a period of time, usually somewhere between 5 and 30 minutes.

However, there are considerable differences between the two approaches. A Western acupuncturist makes a medical diagnosis in the conventional way, uses needles to influence the physiology of the body according to the conventional (scientific) view, and regards the acupuncture as a conventional treatment alongside drugs, surgery or physiotherapy. In contrast, a traditional acupuncturist makes a diagnosis in terms of a disturbance in the body's 'balance' and treatment in terms of its 'correction' with needles.

This chapter includes a brief review of what we know about the physiological mechanisms of acupuncture and how they can provide a rational basis for treating patients. This is intended to be both a summary for the general reader and an introduction for the practitioner, so that the following chapters on mechanisms are more digestible. In this chapter, we avoid technical words where possible, and we keep references to a minimum to avoid distracting the reader.

Acupuncture in the West

Several British doctors discovered the benefits of acupuncture independently, over the last 200 years. Early in the 19th century a London surgeon named John Morse Churchill published two books on acupuncture describing how he treated patients with rheumatic pain by inserting needles into tender points (Baldry, 2005a). A century later, the famous Canadian physician William Osler (1849–1919) discovered acupuncture and recommended inserting hat pins into tender points in the back muscles to treat lumbago. Neither of these eminent doctors used Chinese philosophy to explain acupuncture, but simply inserted needles into the painful points.

The modern history of Western medical acupuncture starts in the 1970s with Felix Mann, a medically qualified doctor who took the trouble to learn Chinese so that he could better understand the acupuncture that he had learned in both Europe and China. The conclusions he drew from his studies and from his clinical experience were quite heretical at the time: 'Meridians don't exist; points don't exist'. This liberated other acupuncturists to think the unthinkable and start to explore a rational approach to acupuncture.

About the same time, research had begun to provide the means to understand the mechanisms of acupuncture. Against the background of the gate control theory of pain (Melzack and Wall, 1965), the discovery of the 'endorphins' (Hughes et al., 1975) was a major advance, followed shortly afterwards by studies that showed that acupuncture released endorphins (Han and Terenius, 1982). This close association between acupuncture and the endorphins, now called 'endogenous opioid peptides', helped enormously to establish the credibility of acupuncture, and this has been reinforced over time by discoveries of other mechanisms of action, as well as by positive clinical trials. Since the 1970s, Western medical acupuncture has gradually earned its place and become more widely accepted alongside conventional Western therapies in modern health service.

Mechanisms for understanding Western medical acupuncture

Western medical acupuncture is based on a contemporary understanding of the body's mechanisms. We have the Chinese to thank for the first scientific investigations of acupuncture and the discovery that acupuncture operates through the nervous system. One crucial experiment in the early days of acupuncture research showed that acupuncture needles had no effect if they were inserted into an area that had been anaesthetized by injection of a local anaesthetic (Chiang et al., 1973). Another early trial showed that acupuncture generates nerve action potentials that can be detected in the nerve trunks leading away from the area being treated (Wang et al., 1985). The great body of research that has accumulated to date leaves little doubt that the majority of acupuncture's effects at different sites of the body are the result of stimulating high-threshold nerves in deep tissue.

LOCAL TISSUE EFFECTS

Acupuncture needles stimulate local nerve endings to release various chemical substances that increase the *blood flow* in the area. This can improve skin conditions and, from an effect in salivary glands, dry mouth. It may improve healing of wounds, and has been used in venous ulcers. Tissue healing might also be aided by the changes that the acupuncture needle causes to fibroblast cells.

Acupuncture releases adenosine locally, directly through tissue injury rather than through nerve stimulation. Adenosine at a relatively low concentration blocks nerves and so causes local analgesia, but higher concentrations from tissue damage are pronociceptive.

More frequently, local acupuncture is used to inactivate trigger points, in particular, those in muscle known as 'myofascial trigger points' (MTrPs). These can arise when a muscle is strained, either in an acute injury or over the longer term by a joint problem or abnormal posture. Small centres of muscle hyperactivity develop where the muscle is dysfunctional, causing pain (Fig 2.1). In many cases these centres correspond with classical acupuncture points. Acupuncture can restore muscle function to normal and reduce or eliminate the pain.

SEGMENTAL EFFECTS

Humans, like all vertebrates, are organized *segmentally* – the spinal cord consists of many segments, each of which is connected to a defined part of the body by nerves, through which it sends and receives information. The activity of each segment changes in response to the input it receives, whether that input comes from the body and organs or from the brain. One of these inputs is

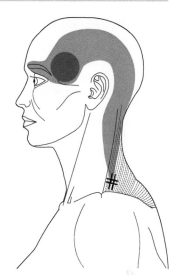

Figure 2.1 Myofascial trigger point in the trapezius muscle causing pain in the neck and head.

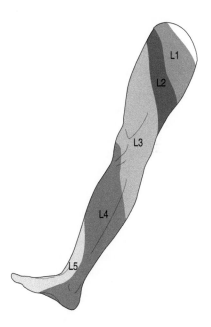

Figure 2.2 Schematic drawing of a leg showing innervation of the skin by different spinal segments. An acupuncture needle reduces pain in the segment which it stimulates.

acupuncture, which can modify the way the spinal cord handles pain signals and the autonomic reflex (Fig 2.2). It can also influence the higher, *supraspinal* centres – particularly in the midbrain and other structures beneath the cortex itself – which influence the function of the spinal segments (i.e. *descending* control). This applies to both pain perception and autonomic control.

In this way, acupuncture affects the function of the segment, both directly and through descending control. This can be effective both in treating pain from structures within the segment and in normalizing the function of organs innervated by the segment, such as bladder and bowel, through the autonomic nervous system.

GENERAL EFFECTS

Treatment with acupuncture influences not only the centres responsible for descending control, but also other brain centres and networks that are responsible for the emotional reactions of the body, for example to pain. The emotional aspect of pain is centred in the *limbic system*, and acupuncture has been shown to modulate its activity, providing important benefits for patients with chronic pain. In addition, the brain's *functional networks* are now known to be disturbed in patients with chronic pain. Again, acupuncture has been shown to help restore the functional networks to normality as the chronic pain resolves.

This link between acupuncture and the functional activity of the brain is interesting and potentially powerful. Acupuncture can be, and must be, distinguished from the placebo response: acupuncture activates some of the pain control mechanisms used by the (equally powerful) placebo response, but there is good evidence that it also uses other networks and pathways (Kong et al., 2009).

Acupuncture is likely to be more than just the sum of the effects of nerve stimulation. To quote an authority on central effects of acupuncture (Napadow et al., 2016),

> *How patients anticipate, perceive and reevaluate acupuncture needling in the context of the patient-practitioner relationship, that is its salience and behavioural relevance are likely to be critical components underlying acupuncture's therapeutic effects. Human research is necessary to answer these questions, and recent applications of neuroimaging to explore acupuncture effects in humans have opened a window to the brain mechanisms supporting both needling and more complex whole treatment effects.*

MECHANISMS NOT YET KNOWN

There are still large gaps in the understanding of the neurophysiology of the human body, but two areas of current research should provide us with an even better understanding of acupuncture mechanisms within the next few years.

Firstly, whilst the mechanisms of chronic pain are incompletely understood, current concepts that are being investigated and show promise include long-term changes in neurotransmitters and their receptors, and the changes to glial cells and the blood–brain barrier.

Secondly, imaging studies, particularly functional magnetic resonance imaging, are revealing the function of the brain and providing a new understanding of the actions of the deeper brain structures, particularly functional networks. These studies have already contributed to a greater understanding of acupuncture.

Additionally, more detail is being discovered about the local effects of acupuncture, and some of these effects may not involve the nervous system directly. For example, evidence is already beginning to accumulate that acupuncture needles may have important effects on connective tissue.

The meaning of Western medical acupuncture

The term 'medical' acupuncture is not meant to imply that only doctors use it, and the words 'modern' or 'scientific' acupuncture would do equally well. They all convey the idea that this approach to acupuncture is based on the current understanding of the structure and function of the body. This is the fundamental difference from the traditional Chinese approach.

The essential features of treatment with Western medical acupuncture are that:

- conventional methods of medical history and examination are used, with clinical investigations if necessary, to establish a conventional diagnosis

- a decision is made on which functions need to be influenced by acupuncture in a particular patient
- the appropriate treatment is given, in a dose that is carefully tailored to the individual
- the treatment is repeated according to the patient's initial response and the changes they report over the subsequent few days.

Western medical acupuncture does not claim to treat every medical condition, nor every individual; acupuncturists need to know when it is appropriate – and when it is inappropriate – to use acupuncture.

Other interpretations of Western medical acupuncture

In this book we describe acupuncture treatment very much in terms of its mechanisms of action. We encourage the acupuncturist to plan a treatment in order to activate the mechanisms that will benefit the patient. This means that our approach is fairly and squarely 'evidence based' – and as a result it will be constantly modified and developed in the light of new research, and become acceptable in an evidence-based health service.

Other approaches to Western acupuncture by respected practitioners focus more on clinical examination and the experience of the practitioner. Mann rejected conventional points in most respects and recommended minimal needling of a restricted number of points (Mann, 1992). Campbell attaches great significance to the patient's reaction to both examination and needling, and uses 'acupuncture treatment areas' rather than traditional points (Campbell, 2001). Both approaches rely heavily on learning by experience, but often the modern practitioner has rather less time to devote to the experimentation and careful observation that are needed to apply these approaches. Macdonald emphasizes the significance of the tender point (Macdonald, 1982), and Baldry, another influential medical acupuncturist, emphasized the treatment of trigger points after the pioneering work of Travell and Simons (Baldry, 1993), and recommended the routine use of superficial needling. Gunn has developed a particular application of acupuncture by concentrating on diagnosis and treatment of radiculopathy, considering this to be the fundamental cause of many cases of chronic pain (Gunn, 1996). He treats the affected segments with deep needling of paravertebral points, a treatment called 'intramuscular stimulation' or IMS.

Other authorities have concentrated on a standardized form of stimulation, particularly electrical stimulation.In Sweden this treatment is called 'sensory stimulation' (Lundeberg, 1999) and in the United States 'scientific acupuncture' (Ulett and Han, 2002).

We recognize and draw on the experience and wisdom of all these experts, and we encourage readers who want to explore all aspects of acupuncture to study their work.

The Western medical approach has been fostered in the UK by the British Medical Acupuncture Society, who aim to 'encourage the scientific understanding' of acupuncture by seeking evidence, rationalizing the treatment approach and distilling its essence into the teaching courses, which have been evolving since the Society's foundation in 1980.

Some schools of thought in acupuncture still cling to the traditional Chinese acupuncture ideology, but add Western physiological understanding to form a kind of hybrid version. Some of these also use the term 'medical acupuncture' (Helms, 1998).

Milestones in Western medical acupuncture

Some of the main contributions to the reevaluation of acupuncture in scientific terms are listed in Table 2.1, although there are countless other clinicians and scientists who have contributed to the critical thinking about acupuncture and have helped to understand it.

TABLE 2.1 ■ Milestones in the development of various aspects of Western medical acupuncture

Date	Name(s)	Topic	Milestone
1952 on	Travell	Myofascial trigger point (MTrP)	Exploration of myofascial origin of pain
1965	Melzack and Wall	Pain concepts	The gate control theory of pain
1973	Chiang et al.	Basic research	Local anaesthetic blocks acupuncture effect
1975	Hughes et al.	Basic research	Discovery of endogenous opioids
1970s on	Han; Pomeranz	Basic research	Acupuncture and neurotransmitter release
1970s on	Mann	Acupuncture concepts	Traditional concepts of acupuncture challenged radically
1977	Melzack	MTrP	Correlation between acupuncture points and myofascial trigger points
1977	Mayer	Basic research	Acupuncture analgesia reversed by naloxone
1980	Clement-Jones	Basic research	Opioid peptides rise in humans after acupuncture
1982	Han and Terenius	Basic research	Classic review article on neurotransmitter release by acupuncture
1980s	Lundeberg	Clinical research	Clinical trials on acupuncture for pain control
1980s	Dundee	Clinical research	Placebo-controlled trials of acupuncture for nausea
1983	Travell and Simons	MTrP	Definitive manual of trigger point therapy published
1992 on	Sato	Basic research	Visceral reflexes
1996 on	Stener-Victorin	Basic and clinical research	Metabolic effects in PCOS
1996	Vickers	Clinical research	First positive systematic review for acupuncture
1997	Gerwin	MTrP	Showed MTrP diagnosis to be reliable
1998 on	Longhurst	Basic research	Cardiovascular reflexes
2000	Hui	Basic research	Effects of acupuncture on the brain showed limbic deactivation by functional magnetic resonance imaging
2006 on	Langevin	Basic research	Effects on connective tissue
2008 on	Kaptchuk	Clinical research	Power of practitioner effect
2012	Vickers	Clinical research	High-quality clinical trials show acupuncture superior to placebo
2007 on	Napadow	Basicand and clinical research	fMRI evidence of effect on brain functional networks

Adapted from Ulett GA. Beyond Yin and Yang: How Acupuncture Really Works. Warren H Green. 1992.

Summary

An acupuncturist using a Western medical approach makes a conventional diagnosis and considers acupuncture as a physiologically based, rational treatment alongside drugs, physical therapy and surgery. The West has flirted with acupuncture at several points in its history, but interest has flourished since it became a plausible treatment with good evidence of neurological effects – mainly its ability to modulate function by releasing neurotransmitters, including the endogenous opioids. Its various known mechanisms can be grouped according to the approach needed to achieve a range of effects – local, segmental and general.

Further reading

Baldry, P., 2005. Acupuncture, Trigger Points and Musculoskeletal Pain. Churchill Livingstone, Edinburgh.

A thorough and detailed textbook that contains valuable information about the development of acupuncture and the modern theory of mechanisms of acupuncture, including extensive acupuncture diagrams of myofascial trigger points.

Campbell, A., 2001. Acupuncture in Practice: Beyond Points and Meridians. Butterworth-Heinemann, Oxford.

A highly readable individual account of medical acupuncture, introducing the idea of an acupuncture treatment area to replace traditional points.

Mann, F., 1992. Reinventing Acupuncture: A New Concept of Ancient Medicine. Butterworth-Heinemann, Oxford.

A personal record by an author who has been at the forefront of Western medical acupuncture, with excellent illustrations as part of an extensive guide to treatment.

CHAPTER 3

Pain, acupuncture and the nervous system

CONTENTS

Introduction

Acupuncture is most commonly used to treat pain. This chapter provides an overview of receptors, pathways and mechanisms of both acupuncture and pain. Though simplified, it aims to provide all the background information that is necessary for understanding the mechanism chapters.

Pain is an unpleasant experience that protects the body by warning of actual or impending damage. The experience is both sensory and emotional and is coloured by one's beliefs, current psychological status and the memory of previous experiences, of one's own pain, and observations of the effects of pain on family and close friends.

An injury does not always cause pain, for example when a person is distracted playing sports. Clearly, the pain signal can be interrupted, or modulated, as it travels from body to brain. This is the essence of the 'gate control theory of pain': there is effectively a 'gate' in the spinal cord which opens or closes to alter the perception of pain in the cerebral cortex. Because a noxious stimulus does not always cause pain, the receptors should be called 'nociceptors' (i.e. receptors of noxious information), and the 'pain pathway' should be called the 'nociceptive pathway'. Figure 3.1 provides a diagrammatic overview of the nociceptive system.

There are different types of pain. In acupuncture practice, we are mainly concerned with nociceptive pain. This covers most chronic musculoskeletal pain, since it results from sensitization of nociceptive pathways, usually through hypoxia (of muscle), inflammation (following damage) or degeneration.

Pain can also be experienced in the absence of either peripheral sensitization or noxious stimulus. This is most commonly *neuropathic* pain, which can occur if the nervous system is itself damaged and malfunctioning, as discussed later.

Pain of purely psychological origin is extremely rare, though every experience of pain includes a psychological dimension. Acupuncture's success in blocking the psychological aspects of pain directly is unpredictable, but it may have other effects that are useful to the patient, such as relaxation and improved sleep. The response to any treatment depends to some extent on the patient's beliefs and expectations and the strength of the therapeutic relationship, as well as any specific effects on the nociceptive pathways. Acupuncture may contribute usefully to recovery of

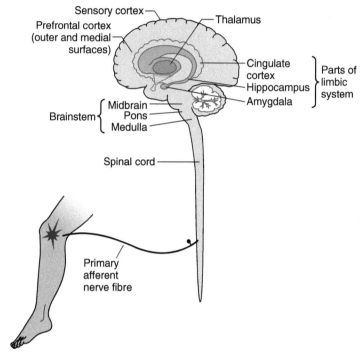

Figure 3.1   Diagram showing main components of pain pathway (viewing brain in midline section).

even severe chronic pain, especially within a pain management strategy that includes information, modification of treatment objectives and exercise.

In a primary-care setting of civilian and military populations (Cummings, 1996), the response rates to acupuncture for different types of pain were as follows:

- 90% in patients with myofascial pain
- 70% in patients with other forms of nociceptive pain
- 40% in other types of pain.

Acute nociceptive pain is often the result of trauma, either accidental or surgical, or of inflammation in arthritis. Pain lasting more than 3–6 months is considered chronic. If severe and prolonged, it may change its nature, causing patients to become depressed and ruminate excessively about their pain.

Pain can be *visceral* or *somatic,* according to its site of origin. Visceral pain arises in the inner organs (e.g. intestinal colic, cystitis). Somatic pain arises mainly in muscles, bones and joints, as well as the skin.

> *Acupuncture is most predictably effective for treating nociceptive pain, especially myofascial pain.*

Receptors

Receptors convert stimuli into electrical signals that alert the brain. We are concerned here with the receptors that are stimulated by noxious stimuli and those stimulated by acupuncture needles.

Different nociceptors can recognize different harms, though *polymodal* receptors respond to all harms, such as strong mechanical stimulation, heat, cold and chemical compounds (e.g. those produced by inflammation). Most nociceptors are a type of mechanoreceptor with a relatively high threshold and are activated by strong pressure. Nociceptors are simply the free endings of certain types of sensory nerve, the C fibre and the Aδ (type III in muscle, see below). These are found throughout somatic tissue (nociception in the viscera is described in a subsequent section).

Acupuncturists usually try to avoid causing pain, aiming to stimulate only the (mechano-) receptors that detect pressure and stretch. These can be either free nerve endings or specialized receptors, such as capsules. These receptors can be located in skin, subcutaneous tissue and muscle, as well as in connective tissue such as ligaments and tendons. Figure 3.2 illustrates the difference

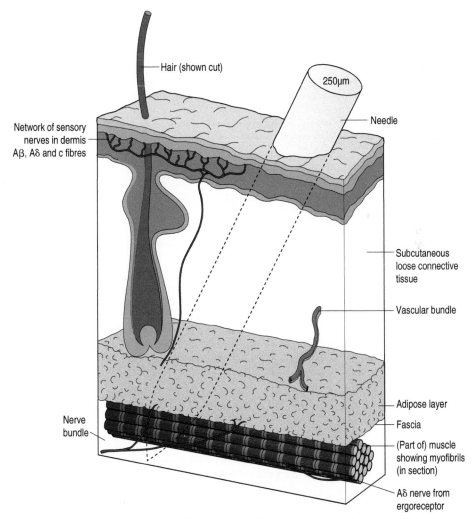

Figure 3.2 Scale diagram of a section of human forearm from skin down to underlying myofibrils, showing relative size of acupuncture needle in situ. Note: Many myofibrils constitute a single muscle fibre. Sensory nerves are too small to be shown to scale.

in scale of these structures in relation to a needle, to indicate how a needle might displace these tissues, applying stretch and pressure. Many of acupuncture's effects are best explained by its stimulating high-threshold pressure receptors in muscle, called 'ergoreceptors' (*ergo* = work). Acupuncture treatment in many ways has effects similar to those of muscular exercise.

So far, we have only discussed acupuncture either without stimulation of needles or with manual stimulation only. In *electroacupuncture* (EA) the nerve fibres are depolarized directly by the current.

Primary afferent nerve fibre

The primary afferent fibre conveys the signal from the receptor to the dorsal horn of the spinal cord (*affero* = bring toward). There are five types of sensory fibre, distinguished by their size and by the thickness of the myelin sheath, which determine the fibre's conducting speed. The three main types that concern us are shown in Table 3.1, which also shows their different names depending on whether they arise in skin or muscle: 'Aβ', 'Aδ' and 'C' fibres from skin, or 'type II', 'III' and 'IV' from muscle.

Just two types of fibre can explain the most about acupuncture (i.e. type III fibres from ergoreceptors in muscle) and about nociception (i.e. C fibres widespread through most tissues). Exceptionally, acupuncture needles may be used to stimulate the nociceptive C fibres of periosteum, a special technique described in Chapter 15.

Aβ/type II fibres convey information from pressure and stretch receptors in skin and connective tissue; they are involved in the related therapy of transcutaneous electrical nerve stimulation (TENS) and also in some of the sensations of needling. The other two types of fibre, Aα and Aγ, convey specialized information from muscle spindles.

Visceral receptor and afferent fibre

Visceral pain is dull and diffuse. If it persists, it becomes referred to the body surface, for example heart pain (angina pectoris) felt in the left arm. Visceral pain often elicits strong reflex autonomic responses, such as sweating and nausea, and can stimulate profound changes of mood.

Visceral pain is caused when mechanoreceptors in the organ wall stretch as the organ distends or when chemoreceptors are stimulated, for example by inflammatory compounds.

The afferent pathways for visceral pain are Aδ fibres and C fibres that travel with sympathetic or parasympathetic nerves. Some afferents terminate in the dorsal horn where they stimulate the autonomic reflex (see Chapter 8); others pass directly up, either via dorsal columns or by the vagus nerve, to nuclei in the brainstem that form the autonomic centre. They also project to the limbic system, where the emotional experience is centred, and to the cortex, where the sensation is felt.

Visceral pain is closely associated with dysfunction of the organ, even if the tissue itself is normal. Irritable bowel and irritable bladder are good examples of this.

TABLE 3.1 ■ **Characteristics of primary afferent nerve fibres**

From skin	From muscle	Diameter	Myelin sheath	Conducting speed
Aβ	Type II	Large	Thick	Fast
Aδ	Type III	Small	Thin	Quite fast
C	Type IV	Small	None	Slow

Dorsal horn of spinal cord: gate control

The essence of the gate control theory of pain (Melzack and Wall, 1965) is that non-nociceptive nerves in an area of the body carry information that reduces the transmission of a local nociceptive stimulus in the dorsal horn. Acupuncture stimulates non-nociceptive nerves, so gate control is the basis of its segmental effect, as described in Chapter 7. We now discuss the gate control mechanism in detail, noting first that 'closing' the gate should be taken to mean reducing the flow through it, not complete closure.

Figure 3.3 reminds the reader of the structure of the spinal cord. Six layers (laminae of Rexid) of nerve cell bodies can be identified in the dorsal horn. For our purposes, we can consider laminae I and II as a pair, laminae III and IV as a pair, and laminae V and VI. The nociceptive fibres and those involved in acupuncture terminate in different layers.

The nociceptive Aδ and C fibres terminate at superficial laminae I-II (also known as 'substantia gelatinosa (SG)') on neurons known as 'SG neurons'. As shown in Figure 3.4, they activate secondary neurons that have a short axon, terminating in lamina V on transmission (T) neurons, which transmit the signal onwards to higher centres (lamina VI seems hardly involved).

The non-nociceptive fibres, including the type III fibres from ergoreceptors stimulated by acupuncture, terminate in laminae III-IV on neurons that pass directly on to higher centres (Fig. 3.5). These non-nociceptive fibres also produce important collateral branches that activate inhibitory intermediate neurons in the substantia gelatinosa, releasing enkephalin, a natural inhibitory opioid peptide that directly inhibits the nociceptive pathway at the SG neuron. In addition, GABA (see Table 3.2 for name in full) is another inhibitor released at this site. Thus type III fibre stimulation inhibits the nociceptive pathway, 'closing the gate' to pain.

Acupuncture 'closes the gate' in the dorsal horn, through release of enkephalin and GABA.

There are two other mechanisms that tend to close the gate. The first is *descending inhibition,* by which information from the midbrain travels downwards to the dorsal horn, releasing transmitters that inhibit the transmission neuron in various ways. This is an important mechanism of acupuncture, discussed in detail in Chapter 9.

And finally, vibration of the skin, or its medical equivalent TENS, stimulates Aβ fibres. These pass directly up the dorsal columns, but also send collaterals into the dorsal horn, which inhibit the nociceptive pathway at the SG neuron.

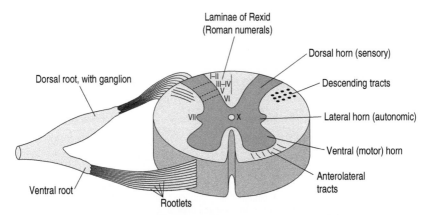

Figure 3.3 Diagrammatic cross-section of spinal cord showing main components of the sensory and autonomic systems. Roman numerals indicate laminae (of Rexid).

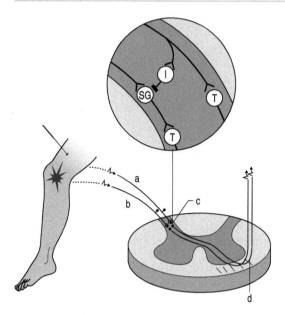

Figure 3.4 Section of spinal cord, showing projections of (a) acupuncture stimulus (myelinated nerve) and (b) noxious stimulus (unmyelinated nerve) to the dorsal horn c. Pathway continues up the anterolateral tract (d). Enlarged section of (c) shows how acupuncture stimulus can suppress the response of the SG neuron leading to inhibition of pain. Key: SG = substantia gelatinosa neuron. T = transmission neuron. I = intermediate neuron (inhibitory).

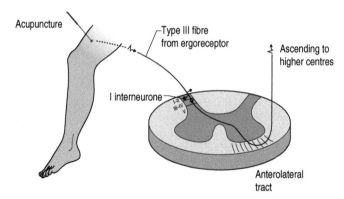

Figure 3.5 Non-nociceptive pathways. Diagram of dorsal horn showing pathways of non-nociceptive fibres, including type III from ergoreceptors stimulated by the acupuncture needle. A collateral branch projects onto an inhibitory interneuron (I), which inhibits the nociceptive pathway.

TABLE 3.2 ▧ **The main neurotransmitters (short-term effect) and neuromodulators (longer-term effect) involved in the sensory pathway**

	Excitatory	Inhibitory
Sensory nerve ending	Bradykinin	Adenosine
	Substance P (SP)	
	Serotonin (5HT)	
Dorsal horn	Glutamate (GLU)	Glycine (GLY)
	Substance P (SP)	γ-aminobutyric acid (GABA)
	Serotonin (5HT)	Enkephalin
	Calcitonin gene-related peptide	Noradrenalin
	(CGRP) [releases GLU and SP]	

The transmitters involved in excitation and inhibition are shown in Table 3.2, for reference. In general, nociceptive fibres release excitatory transmitters GLU and SP. Type III fibres and interneurons inhibit directly by releasing the endogenous opioid peptide enkephalin and indirectly by GLY and GABA.

Afferent signals from viscera also terminate in the dorsal horn onto neurons that project directly to lamina VII (Fig. 3.6). Lamina VII is known as the 'lateral horn' and contains the motor or efferent (*effere* = carry away) neurons of the autonomic system. In this way, the incoming signals stimulate reflex changes in autonomic outflow. Acupuncture can influence the autonomic reflex at the dorsal horn (see Chapter 8).

Ascending spinal pathway and higher centres

From the dorsal horn, the nociceptive and acupuncture pathways cross and ascend to the higher centres in the anterolateral tract (also called 'spinothalamic tract', since many fibres terminate in the thalamus).

Two aspects of pain can be readily separated: sensory/discriminatory (awareness) and affective/motivational (suffering) (Melzack and Wall, 1988). The brain deals with them differently. This distinction is relevant to us, since acupuncture often seems to influence the affective component more than the sensation of pain: 'The pain is still there but does not bother me so much'.

The sensory/discriminative component (the intensity, location, quality and duration of the pain) is the function of the majority of fibres in the anterolateral tract. They project to the thalamus and then directly to the sensory cortex (both primary and secondary cortices).

The affective/motivational (the unpleasantness and urge to escape) component stimulates various areas of the cortex and some subcortical centres, together known as the 'limbic system'. The limbic system receives input from the anterolateral tract via the reticular formation in the brainstem. It links to all parts of the brain: especially relevant to us are its links to the hypothalamus (for hormone control), through the hypothalamus to the autonomic centre (for autonomic regulation), and to the default mode network (see next page, and Chapter 10). Acupuncture has been shown to modulate the activity of the limbic system to a significant degree compared with sham acupuncture, and this effect is discussed more fully in Chapter 10.

There remains a small but important group of fibres in the anterolateral tract, which project to the periaqueductal grey matter (PAG), in the midbrain. The PAG has many opioid receptors and is an important centre for pain control. Both nociceptive and type III fibres stimulate the

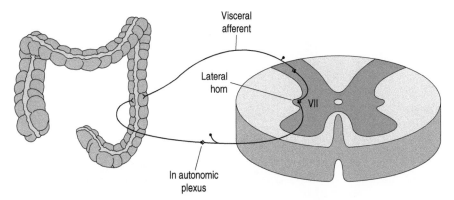

Figure 3.6 Spinal autonomic reflex. Diagram of dorsal horn between T1 and L2 and the large intestine, showing a visceral afferent nerve synapsing in the dorsal horn and projecting onto the cell body of the autonomic efferent in the lateral grey horn (lamina VII).

release of β endorphin in the PAG, triggering descending pain inhibition. Tracts descend to every level of the spinal cord, releasing serotonin, which activates the inhibitory interneurons releasing met-enkephalin or noradrenaline, which diffuses through the dorsal horn. Both met-enkephalin and noradrenaline have the effect of diminishing the firing of nociceptive neurons. Descending pain inhibition is an important means of pain control that will be discussed in relation to acupuncture at several points in this book and also has its own chapter (Chapter 9).

Brain imaging reveals that each area of the brain has its own slow, regular fluctuation of activity and that the activity of two or three areas can fluctuate in precise synchrony, making functional networks. One network particularly relevant to pain and acupuncture is the default mode network (DMN), consisting of three cortical areas that are synchronous when resting quietly. Chronic pain has been linked to disturbances of the DMN, and some early studies of acupuncture have shown it can modulate the DMN. The improvement in the DMN in different individuals over a course of acupuncture correlates with their improvement in back pain scores.

Functional connectivity is very interesting and might explain the higher level mechanisms of acupuncture in treatment of chronic pain patients.

Sensitization: peripheral and central

In certain circumstances, a patient's response to a noxious stimulus can be amplified out of proportion to the apparent degree of injury or pathology. For example, an inflamed joint may be extremely tender to the lightest touch, or a limb that has recovered from injury may remain unduly sensitive. This sensitization can be either peripheral or central.

- Peripheral sensitization: the sensory nerve endings are sensitized by inflammatory mediators released locally, such as neuropeptides, cytokines and nitric oxide (NO). The immune response is also involved, and mast cells and macrophages are found adjacent to nociceptors. Primary hyperalgesia (excessive pain response to a painful stimulus) and allodynia (pain caused by a normally painless stimulus like brushing the skin or light touch) occurs within a segment or two above and below the stimulus, but not throughout the body.
- Central sensitization: a form of amplification of electrical signals in neurons within the CNS – principally in the spinal cord. It results in secondary hyperalgesia and allodynia. The size of the neuronal receptive fields is increased. It is the result of several mechanisms in dorsal horn and higher centres, including for example the opening of receptors that are normally silent, as shown in Figure 3.7.

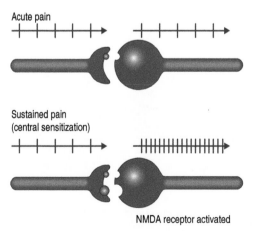

Acute pain

Sustained pain
(central sensitization)

NMDA receptor activated

Figure 3.7 Schematic drawing of central sentization, showing the standard response of the pathway to acute pain and the heightened response in chronic pain when the second receptor is activated.

■ If a nociceptive stimulus is repeated, the response of some spinal cord transmission cells increases, which is a normal physiological form of central sensitization called 'wind up' (Woolf, 1996). When this becomes abnormally prolonged or severe it is referred to as central sensitization.

Tenderness throughout the body may indicate central sensitization, or in fibromyalgia a deficit in tonic descending inhibition.

Neuropathic pain

Neuropathic pain is caused by injury or dysfunction of the nervous system itself. Attacks of pain may occur spontaneously or may consist of highly amplified responses to minor stimulation. Well-recognized examples include postherpetic neuralgia, phantom limb pain, poststroke pain and complex regional pain syndrome. Other causes include infections (e.g. HIV), chemotherapy, radiotherapy and diabetes. Patients often describe neuropathic pain with characteristic adjectives ('shooting' or 'burning'), and they may have allodynia and hyperalgesia. Since the nervous system is itself damaged, it is hardly surprising that acupuncture is sometimes less helpful for patients with neuropathic pain. In addition, there is a risk that acupuncture will exacerbate neuropathic pain if it is not performed carefully.

Other aspects of nociception

Nociception can involve other cells in the CNS apart from the neurons. Astrocytes and other microglia, the central counterparts of peripheral immune cells and connective tissue cells, may be activated in chronic pain states. There is some early evidence that acupuncture can influence these cells, but not yet enough to inform clinical application.

Outside the nervous system, manipulating an acupuncture needle can activate the fibroblasts in the connective tissue, some distance away from the needle. This causes changes that may be therapeutic, as discussed in Chapter 5.

Summary

Different types of pain may arise from different noxious stimuli, not all of which respond to acupuncture treatment. Some nociceptors respond to deep pressure, others to a variety of stimuli, including the chemicals released by inflammation. Acupuncture's main effects arise from stimulation of high-threshold receptors that detect the work done by the muscle – ergoreceptors. Much of acupuncture's effect on pain is obtained by 'closing the gate to pain' in the dorsal horn of the spinal cord both by direct reflex effect and by activating descending inhibitory systems. Acupuncture can also have profound effects on central processes within the brain.

Further reading

Gupta, R., Farquhar-Smith, P., 2016. Neurophysiology of chronic pain. In: Filshie, J., White, A., Cummings, M. (Eds.), Medical Acupuncture: A Western Scientific Approach, second ed. Elsevier, Edinburgh, pp. 73–85.
    A detailed description of pain pathways and pain neurophysiology.
Melzack, R., Wall, P.D., 1988. The Challenge of Pain. Penguin Books, London.
    The classic, but still eminently readable, text on pain gate theory.

Lundeberg, T., Lund, I., 2016. Peripheral components of acupuncture stimulation – their contribution to the specific clinical effects of acupuncture. In: Filshie, J., White, A., Cummings, M. (Eds.), Medical Acupuncture: A Western Scientific Approach, second ed. Elsevier, Edinburgh, pp. 22–58.

A detailed discussion of the effects of acupuncture upon the nervous system.

Reddi, D., Curran, N.H. An introduction to pain pathways and mechanisms. www.ucl.ac.uk/anaesthesia/StudentsandTrainees/PainPathwaysIntroduction. (Accessed February 2017).

A short but highly accessible summary of the neurophysiology of pain.

An introduction to acupuncture technique

Introduction

Acupuncture techniques have evolved over centuries through observation, trial and error – and sometimes in order to promote a particular training school! We have inherited many varied and often implausible idiosyncratic treatment methods. One of the tasks of Western medical acupuncture is to apply research and critical thinking to re-evaluate treatment suitable for a modern health service.

This chapter aims to provide an introduction to using acupuncture techniques to generate changes in the body. It provides a background for making sense of the chapters on mechanisms; more detailed advice on technique is given in Chapter 15.

An acupuncturist will want to have a clear idea of the *aim* of treatment, as this will determine the location and type of stimulation and answer questions such as:

- Where should I place the needles?
- How many needles?
- How deep?
- How should I stimulate them?
- What sensation should be achieved?
- How long should the needle be retained?
- What constitutes a course of treatment?

Many of acupuncture's benefits are the result of inhibitory effects in the central nervous system (CNS), not excitatory effects. Treatment must be rather carefully judged to achieve the inhibition without any excess irritation, as not all responses will be therapeutic.

This chapter assumes readers are familiar with the pain and acupuncture pathways discussed in the previous chapter.

A typical acupuncture stimulus

The most significant part of acupuncture treatment seems to be when the needles are inserted into muscle and stretch and press the muscle fibres, activating ergoreceptors and generating signals in type III fibres.

This stimulation effect might be amplified if the muscle itself contracts. Manual rotation of the needle may activate reflex muscle contraction, which activates ergoreceptors further and also activates stretch-sensitive free endings in the muscle and tendon, at least for points near the ends of muscle. This all adds to stimulation of the type III fibres.

We present a typical case report here to introduce readers to the general approach to acupuncture. This treatment could be considered typical but should not be regarded as a standard because nothing in acupuncture should be standardized – except safety. Every patient is treated individually according to the acupuncturist's clinical evaluation.

Electroacupuncture

Electroacupuncture (EA) involves running a small electrical current between two needles, using a dedicated apparatus. EA depolarizes nerve fibres directly (i.e. not through receptors). Large nerve fibres have a lower electrical threshold than small fibres, meaning they are fired off by a smaller current. Thus low-intensity EA will be felt as tingling in the skin and may stimulate motor nerves, causing contraction of the whole muscle; higher intensity will stimulate muscle fibres directly and cause muscle contraction in a smaller area; and still higher intensity stimulates the smallest fibres (i.e. nociceptive C fibres) which may cause pain, and so should be avoided.

Case Report

A 30-year-old mother of two small children presents with right-sided low back pain for 6 weeks. She believes it is caused by lifting her children, and she recalls having a similar pain during her second pregnancy which was relieved by yoga. She has no other relevant history, in particular no rheumatic disease and no cancer.

Examination reveals tender spasms of the right lumbar muscles but little else, and no focal tenderness. There are no 'red flag' symptoms or signs to indicate significant pathology. She is therefore offered acupuncture to achieve some pain relief that will allow her to stretch and exercise her back, and she is encouraged at the same time to pay attention to her lifting techniques.

There are no contraindications to acupuncture; it is a valid approach for her condition. The practitioner is confident that he/she has the knowledge and skill to apply acupuncture and deal with any adverse effects, and that the patient does not need further investigation.

The patient has not had acupuncture before, so we do not know how strongly she will react. With the patient lying on her left side, three needles are inserted into the muscles of the lumbar region and gently manipulated for about 5 seconds each. Needles are removed after 10 minutes, and the sites are checked for bleeding.

The patient returns the following week, saying her pain was relieved for the rest of the day but recurred the next day; she had no adverse reaction to treatment, and she has restarted her yoga. The demands of childcare are making her somewhat tense. Muscle spasm is still present, with no focal tenderness that might suggest a trigger point. For her second treatment, the same three sites are needled, and additional needles are inserted into a point on the forefoot (called 'LR3') on both sides, aiming to both relieve the pain and help her relax. All needles are manipulated and left for 20 minutes.

The following week, she phones to cancel her next appointment as she feels much relieved, is sleeping better and is being more careful with her lifting.

Both MA and EA can sometimes cause excruciating sharp pain – probably when the needle touches the *nervi vasorum*. The needle must be withdrawn straightaway, at least partially, to resolve the pain.

Sensation of *de qi*

Acupuncture needles may produce a needle sensation that the Chinese called '*de qi*'. This sensation was traditionally described as having four components (Lu and Needham, 1980):
- numbness
- distension/extension/fullness
- heaviness
- sour ache 'like a feeling of muscular fatigue'.

Patients also describe the sensations of pressure, tingling, warmth or cold, and the spreading or radiation of sensations (Hui et al., 2000; Vincent et al., 1989). These *de qi* sensations can usually be identified separately from the sensations of simply being pricked with a needle – sharpness or pain. Patients may feel either or both, but it is the *de qi* sensation that is peculiar to acupuncture and a mark that the correct nerve endings have been successfully stimulated.

Nerve conduction studies have shown that the onset of *de qi* is accompanied by action potentials that both travel at the speed and have the waveform appearance, typical of stimulation of Aδ fibres (Wang et al., 1985). In addition, the aching, heavy sensation of *de qi* is comparable to the deep muscle ache after exercise (Andersson and Lundeberg, 1995) that arises from stimulation of the free endings of type II/III fibres (thought to be ergoreceptor fibres).

The arrival of the sensation *de qi* was interpreted in traditional Chinese medicine as indicating 'the gathering of the *qi*', the event that is necessary in producing a response. This is not so very far away from our interpretation according to current Western medical concepts – *de qi* is taken as an indication that the appropriate nerves are being stimulated.

Rather confusingly, the term '*de qi*' is also used to describe the sensation the practitioner feels when the tissues seem to grab the acupuncture needle as it is rotated to and fro in the point, though this is less likely when using modern, highly polished needles.

Evidence suggests numbness, distension and heaviness are mediated by Aβ and Aδ fibres, and aching or soreness by Aδ and C fibres.

There is some evidence that *de qi* is associated with improved outcome (e.g. Spaeth et al., 2013). However, in clinical practice patients often improve when *de qi* is not being elicited – either intentionally or because it is impossible.

Where to place the needle?

Local effects can be obtained by needling almost anywhere, but there also exist, throughout the body, certain sites that have come to be regarded as especially effective – some of the classical 'acupuncture points'.

From the practical point of view, it is useful to think of three types of point location, depending on which effect the patient requires: *local, segmental* and *general*. We should be clear that any needle may have effects in all three categories, even if only one effect is needed.

ACUPUNCTURE POINTS

Acupuncture points are a rather obvious and well-known feature of acupuncture. They are usually thought of as the recognized sites that are described in books and on anatomical charts. According to authoritative sources, there are 361 points, mostly arranged in 'meridians', which can be seen on charts (The Academy of Traditional Chinese Medicine, 1975).

This gives the impression that acupuncture points are precise, fixed locations on which everybody agrees, but this is actually far from true. Acupuncture students who have just been trained in college do not agree where the points are. Even the experienced lecturers in acupuncture who taught one of the authors at a recognized college disagreed over the precise location of some points. There is no objective test for points, such as temperature change or electrical skin resistance. Research into acupuncture points has not revealed any unique receptor or other structure for the acupuncture needle to activate. However, some points show an increased density of nerve endings, at least in animal studies, and some points are clearly associated with trigger points in muscle, or lie over deep nerve trunks. Also, brain imaging sometimes shows different responses from verum and sham points that have been needled in the same way, suggesting that at least some points have specific characteristics.

The precise locations of acupuncture points are not as reliable as tradition suggests.

Our approach is this. We think it is helpful for acupuncturists to learn a number of classical points for several reasons: acupuncture points are convenient locations where it is usually easy to elicit a good *de qi* sensation; some points appear repeatedly in formulae for treating a wide variety of conditions, probably because they have rather general neurological effects – we call these the 'well-known' points (another term is 'major' points); and other points are useful because they are used to treat common conditions. In addition, it is convenient to keep the names of the acupuncture points as they provide a reasonably consistent way to report where you inserted the needle, both for keeping a record and for reporting in papers or discussing with other practitioners.

However, Western medical acupuncturists need not worry about the precise location of these points to the nearest millimetre. Learn the rough location, then use the fingertip either to find maximal tenderness or to identify a dip in the tissues. Experienced practitioners of Western medical acupuncture generally find they use a limited number of classical points – the well-known points – repeatedly, and then they use other locations that are tender.

A small number of well-known points can be used in classical formulae for treating many different conditions.

NUMBERING SYSTEM OF ACUPUNCTURE POINTS

We continue to use the classical numbering for acupuncture points simply because there is no other accepted scheme. On the classical charts, points are placed on *meridians,* some of which correspond with fascial planes, while most are not physical structures. Most meridians are named after an organ of the body, such as 'Liver' or 'Gall Bladder'. All the points on each meridian are numbered in sequence; however, inconveniently, the meridians are not all numbered in the same direction! The standard abbreviation for a point consists of two capital letters – for example, 'LU', 'LI' and 'ST' – and a number. The letters stand for 'Lung', 'Large Intestine' and 'Stomach' respectively, so typical points are labelled 'LU7', 'LI4' and 'ST36' (see Tables 19.6 and 19.7 for full list). This is the nomenclature that has been established by international convention and that we shall use throughout this book. Unfortunately for anyone learning acupuncture, other authorities use different nomenclature systems.

The names of the meridians have nothing to do with the actual internal organs, as far as we know. In written text, it is easy to distinguish between 'Liver' as the meridian and 'liver' as the organ. But when you are talking to patients, they are naturally very interested when you say you are going to treat 'Liver 3' or 'Gall Bladder 34', for example. They may even tend to assume there is something wrong with their actual liver or gall bladder and thus need an explanation.

Annoyingly, some points that are quite useful today were only introduced long after the original charts were defined, so they had to be labelled as 'Extra points'. These are usually referred to by their *Pinyin* names, without any numbers. We shall come across an example of this with two useful points on the face (*Yintang* and *Taiyang*), as well as a whole line of points close to the thoracic and lumbar spine, the *Huatuojiaji* (pronounced 'hwa-two-oh-cha-chi') points.

Even more annoyingly, there are different versions of the sequence of numbers in one meridian, Bladder (BL). One system numbers down to the knee before returning to the top of the back and descending again; the other system reaches the sacrum then turns back up before descending again. Both systems use the same numbering below the knee.

> *The classical numbering for acupuncture points is still used as a convenient convention.*

Needle stimulation: the acupuncture 'dose'

The overall amount of stimulation you give the patient may be more significant than the exact locations where it is given. This is the 'dose' of acupuncture, and it depends on several factors, like the number of points treated at a time, the depth of needling and the strength of stimulation. Because there has been little research into these different factors, we are still unsure about the contribution each of them makes to the total dose of a treatment. However, empirically, it is important to be able to vary the dose to suit the patient and the condition, and we shall repeatedly return to this subject throughout the book. Here we shall summarize the main factors and then the way they can be combined into what we might regard as a typical acupuncture treatment.

STRONG RESPONDERS

Patients vary considerably in their response to acupuncture. A small percentage of patients respond to acupuncture –in terms of both benefits and adverse effects – much more strongly than most. They respond well to brief, superficial needling and may experience ill effects from any stronger treatment. This should always be born in mind when thinking about 'dose', and it is discussed more thoroughly in Chapter 15. Other patients fail to respond to even strong, prolonged stimulation and are classified as 'non-responders'. The majority of the population lies somewhere in between these two extremes and responds in a way that we can recognize as 'normal'.

This variation in response is likely to be due to differences in patients' central nervous system, such as opioid peptide metabolism and receptor activity. In laboratory experiments, genetic differences between individual animals of the same species can cause up to 50% of some batches of animals to fail to respond to needling stimulation in the expected way. So it is likely that genetic differences among humans explain their different responses.

NUMBER OF NEEDLES

The appropriate dose of acupuncture may require insertion of a single needle or up to about 20. However, as a general rule, we advise only using up to about six needles for the initial treatment to observe the response. This may be enough to achieve a response, because some patients seem very sensitive to acupuncture.

NEEDLE THICKNESS (DIAMETER)

Clinical experience seems to support the intuitive concept that thicker needles (larger diameter of the shaft) provide stronger stimulation, which may simply be due to the fact that they are stiffer and exert more pressure when they are manipulated.

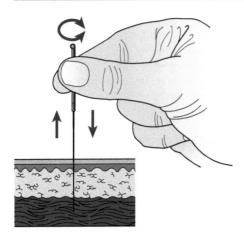

Figure 4.1 Two methods of manipulating a needle to elicit *de qi*.

DEPTH OF INSERTION

We favour needling into muscle belly as the basic technique for the purposes of this book, even though many acupuncturists only needle the skin and subcutaneous tissues. For example, Japanese acupuncturists use superficial needling for many conditions, and some medical acupuncturists generally prefer to use superficial needling for myofascial trigger points (Baldry, 2005b; Macdonald, 1982). It may be less easy to achieve the full-blown *de qi* phenomenon with superficial needling, though there is no doubt that some sensations can occur.

NEEDLE MANIPULATION TO ELICIT *DE QI*

The *de qi* sensation may occur spontaneously after the needle has been inserted, but often the acupuncturist needs to elicit it actively by stimulating the needle. It is generally enough to rotate the needle between finger and thumb, but it may be necessary to include an up-and-down movement as well, sometimes called 'sparrow-pecking' (Fig. 4.1). In this way, the needle reaches enough nerves to generate *de qi*. Quite often, the acupuncturist will feel a tightening of the tissues or needle grasp at about the same time as the patient experiences *de qi*, although this happens less with smoothly polished needles.

Clinical experience and some evidence suggests that patients who feel *de qi* are more likely to respond to the treatment.

One thing is clear: there is no need to treat so vigorously that C fibres are stimulated, causing pain. Acupuncture can be effective without being unpleasant or aversive. It has to be admitted that some Chinese acupuncturists treat their patients strongly, but cultural differences may be relevant, and in the West painful treatment may be counterproductive. If a patient needs stronger stimulation, then in most situations it is preferable to use electrical stimulation than to manipulate the needles very forcefully.

Acupuncture does not need to be painful.

NEEDLE RETENTION TIME

The time that the needles should be left in place depends somewhat on the desired effect. It takes 20–30 minutes to achieve acute analgesia with EA, for example. Some effects (autonomic

TABLE 4.1 ■ **Ranges available for the various parameters of acupuncture treatment**

Parameter	Range
Number of points used	1–20
Depth of insertion	Superficial (subcutaneous); muscle or deep connective tissue; periosteum[a]
Needle stimulation	Manipulation: none; mild; strong. Electroacupuncture (EA)
Sensation elicited	None; de qi; tolerable discomfort. With EA: muscle contraction; tolerable discomfort
Needle retention time	5 seconds to 30 minutes

[a]Periosteal acupuncture is a special technique (see Chapter 15).

modulation, for example) can be obtained after 10 minutes or so, and myofascial trigger points can be inactivated without keeping the needle in place at all.

These times are not hard and fast; they should be altered according to the patient's response, and some acupuncturists find they can obtain results with as little as 30 seconds' needling. At the other extreme, needles can be left for 1 hour or more, for example to reduce pain in the postoperative period. For many patients in clinical practice, there is probably not much difference between the effects of retaining the needles for a few minutes compared with half an hour, provided that the patient does not have specific expectations about treatment time.

TYPICAL TREATMENT 'DOSE'

A typical range of treatment parameters is described in Table 4.1. Each of the variables can be adjusted to take into account the patient's medical condition, general physical condition, immediate responses during needling and (in subsequent treatments) the symptom changes reported in the hours and days following needling. Typical examples of the ranges for the various parameters are given in Table 4.1.

Care and skill are needed to give the right dose of acupuncture.

Cumulative response to acupuncture

In treating many painful conditions with acupuncture, relief of pain usually accumulates gradually over a series of treatments. This may be explained by neuroplasticity: repeated treatments induce changes in genetic expression of transmitters and receptors. For example, a stimulus that leads to the release of opioid peptides also enhances gene expression so that more opioid peptide is manufactured and stored at the terminal; next time the stimulus is applied, it releases more peptide. This increased gene expression needs to be reinforced within a short period of time, or it will decay back to normal. The optimal interval may be about 3 days initially, although in clinical practice it is often difficult to arrange treatments this frequently.

The effect of acupuncture accumulates when it is repeated.

Summary

Acupuncture treatment involves giving a particular stimulus to one or more particular sites. The details of stimulus and site are determined according to the effect intended on the patient's diagnosis. The dose of the stimulus can be varied according to the number of needles as well as their depth and degree of stimulation. The needles may produce a unique sensation known as '*de qi*', which may indicate that active treatment is underway. This book uses classical acupuncture point names as a convenient convention, though each point's effects are not as specific as traditionally believed, and nerves may be stimulated effectively almost anywhere in the body.

Effects Mechanisms Techniques

CHAPTER 5

Local effects I: analgesia, increased blood flow

Introduction

This section of the book deals with effects and mechanisms, starting with effects local to the needling site, then working outwards to more distant effects. The treatment described in this first chapter actually does not play a large part in typical acupuncture practice, although the effects can be important in specific cases and should be understood. The main mechanisms we shall discuss are increased blood flow and local analgesia.

Pain relief from acupuncture is routinely called 'analgesia'. But 'analgesia' is used here loosely, in the sense of reduction of pain, not abolition as in the strict sense. The same applies to drugs called 'analgesics'. This loose usage has probably arisen because the more accurate term, 'hypoalgesia', is clumsy and less well known. Acupuncture often reduces pain, but less often abolishes it completely.

Increased blood flow

It is common to see erythema around the needle site, indicating increased local blood flow (see Plate 3). Sometimes, this is a full-blown wheal-and-flare reaction. Erythema is particularly visible on the trunk, but the increased blood flow occurs equally in deeper tissues such as muscles when the needles penetrate more deeply. The blood flow to the skin and muscle of healthy volunteers increases as soon as a needle is inserted into the skin, increases further when the needle is advanced into the underlying muscle, and increases still further when the needle is stimulated and *de qi* elicited (Sandberg et al., 2003).

This is an example of an 'axon reflex', which occurs when a stimulus spreads around the terminal branches of a nerve. The effects are purely local and do not depend on the dorsal horn.

When a sensory nerve is activated mechanically, it releases a number of neuropeptides, one of which is calcitonin gene-related peptide (CGRP). This peptide increases blood flow in the short term and the long term by several mechanisms. In the short term, CGRP binds to the cell wall of capillaries, causing the smooth muscle to relax, which means vasodilation. CGRP also binds to receptors on the vascular endothelium, triggering production of nitric oxide (NO); NO also relaxes the vascular smooth muscle, reinforcing the vasodilation. CGRP stimulates new blood vessel formation (angiogenesis), causing longer term increases in blood flow. This may improve healing rates.

Furthermore, adenosine is released from various local tissues by acupuncture stimulation (see the next section, Local analgesia); adenosine has vasodilatory effects of its own, as well as stimulating the release of NO.

Needling also releases into the surrounding area other neuropeptides that stimulate vasodilation. Substance P (SP), released in response to stress, is an excitatory molecule with receptors on many different kinds of tissues and is involved in the wheal-and-flare reaction. Nerve growth factor (NGF) has many effects, including acceleration of wound healing, and is released by acupuncture.

The increased blood flow, together with the release of a variety of other mediators, can have other useful clinical effects. Local skin conditions may respond, as may local tissue such as dysfunctional salivary glands. Patients with dry mouth due to postirradiation xerostomia recorded an increase in saliva production and a reduction of symptoms, after acupuncture at local points around the salivary glands. Anecdotal evidence suggests the long-term effects of angiogenesis from CGRP can improve healing of venous ('varicose') ulcers of the leg.

Local analgesia

Research in human subjects shows reliably that acupuncture has analgesic effects superior to sham acupuncture. In particular, acupuncture inhibits deep pressure to a clinically significant degree, which is considered a good model of musculoskeletal pain.

There are several mechanisms for this analgesia. Here we discuss a purely local effect, greatest at the site of needling, which is due to local release of *adenosine* from local cells. Adenosine blocks C fibres (Goldman et al., 2010). Other mechanisms of analgesia occur at other levels – segmental analgesia (Chapter 7) and descending inhibition (Chapter 9).

Adenosine is released locally from various cells, including fibroblasts, by the mild tissue damage caused by acupuncture needles. This extracellular adenosine binds to the cell walls of nociceptors and inhibits their response to stimulation.

In clinical practice, it tends to be enthusiasts who use this local analgesia effect in particular settings, for example, in accident and emergency settings. Anaesthetists who use acupuncture to reduce the dose of analgesic drugs may apply local acupuncture around the incision site, as well as needling other locations for more general effects.

Connective tissue effects

Loose connective tissue consisting of collagen fibres and fibroblasts is present in the locations that are needled, and the response to acupuncture has been investigated by Langevin and colleagues (Langevin et al., 2001, 2006).

Twisting of needles causes deformation of the surrounding tissue, reaching at least 25 mm. This changes the internal structure of fibroblasts. This could be just a mechanical effect, or it could also be the effect of release of adenosine (and the related compounds) by the tissue injury from the needle (Goldman et al., 2013). The changes seen in the fibroblasts could affect their role in regulating tension in the local connective tissue, which in turn may be relevant to the healing of chronic soft tissue injuries.

Inflammation

C fibres can be stimulated by strong, painful acupuncture (not recommended for beginners as it may produce reactions), leading to the release of CGRP as mentioned previously, as well as release of substance P (SP), which causes leakiness of blood vessels. C fibre stimulation can generate *neurogenic inflammation*, that is, increased blood flow and extravasation of fluid (i.e. oedema). It is not yet clear whether this mechanism is useful in clinical practice.

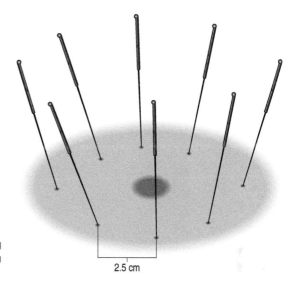

Figure 5.1 Needles surrounding a local skin lesion, a treatment known as 'fencing in the dragon'.

2.5 cm

Cytokine release

Acupuncture can stimulate local release of cytokines (NGF, PGE2) that communicate with the local immune cells. These may be involved in neuroprotective effects that have been attributed to acupuncture, but currently this is best regarded as a useful added effect rather than a mechanism that can be reliably induced.

Clinical application

Three different forms of acupuncture can be useful for different types of local response – superficial skin conditions, deep vascular lesions such as ulcers, and analgesia.

For superficial skin conditions (aiming to use a combination of improved blood flow, immune modulation and inflammatory responses), simply insert a few needles close to the area where the local changes are needed. This could be useful for a lesion that is slow to heal, for example. It may be convenient to surround the area with a ring of needles about 25 mm apart (since the axon reflex covers a 25 mm radius). This treatment was known picturesquely by the Chinese as 'fencing in the dragon' (see Fig. 5.1).

For longer-term pathology such as a venous ulcer, treatment has been described using EA across the ulcer, attached to needles on either side (Yue et al., 2013). Anecdotally, others have used several pairs of needles around the periphery of the ulcer, though the authors do not have personal experience of this. Be careful to insert the needles only into healthy skin with an intact nerve supply.

For acute analgesia, needling down to muscle is likely to be needed, with at least some manual stimulation adding EA for operative analgesia.

Summary

Acupuncture may increase blood flow locally by a variety of mechanisms, an effect which can aid tissue healing. Acupuncture can reduce pain in the area close to the needles; this is commonly called 'analgesia' but should more strictly be called 'hypalgesia'. This effect is largely achieved by release of adenosine from needled tissues.

CHAPTER 6

Local effects II: myofascial trigger point inactivation

CONTENTS

Introduction

One of the oldest maxims in traditional acupuncture is to 'place the needle where the pain is'. The most precise form of this practice involves the practitioner examining a muscle to find its most tender point and needling that exact point. He or she then stimulates the needle and may withdraw it straightaway. Sometimes, the patient experiences immediate relief of pain. In our experience, acupuncture is most rapidly effective for a particular type of tender point called a 'myofascial trigger point' (MTrP). It is not unreasonable to speculate that acupuncture may have been developed originally as a treatment for these MTrPs.

Muscles form the largest organ in the body. They usually recover rapidly from injury, but occasionally they develop a tender and hyperirritable spot, the MTrP. This can cause persistent pain, which has certain characteristics that can help distinguish it from other painful conditions. This chapter discusses the MTrP rather thoroughly, as it is rarely part of the medical curriculum.

The two authors who have made the greatest contribution to the understanding of trigger points are Travell and Simons (Simons et al., 1999; Travell and Simons, 1983, 1992). Their rigorous approach to the diagnosis, mechanisms and treatment of the MTrP syndrome established it as a clinical condition separate from a confusing rag-bag of doubtful or non-committal diagnoses in soft-tissue pain disorders, such as fibrositis, myalgia and muscular or non-articular rheumatism.

Many conventional healthcare practitioners are unfamiliar with the MTrP and have difficulty accepting it as a condition. Even physicians specializing in orthopaedics or rheumatology often dismiss MTrP pain, even though it must be common in the type of patients they see. The whole subject of soft-tissue pain may be seen as a 'grey area' of borderline diagnoses and dismissed as 'functional'.

There is now considerable accumulated clinical experience in treating the MTrP, and the evidence in support of the MTrP as a genuine clinical entity is marked by the following milestones:

- Pain arising from muscles often has a referred component. In an extensive series of experiments, Kellgren injected himself and his colleagues with hypertonic saline and mapped out the resulting pain referral patterns, which were perceived to be similar to clinically relevant pain in nature and distribution. Injections into most soft tissues produced local pain, but injections into muscle consistently caused pain to be referred at a distance (Kellgren, 1938). This has been amply confirmed in many studies since that time.
- MTrPs generate spontaneous electrical activity of greater amplitude than normal muscle (Hubbard and Berkoff, 1993).
- The diagnosis of MTrPs can be made reliably by blinded examiners – if they are appropriately trained (Gerwin et al., 1997).
- A hypothesis for a mechanism has been proposed (Mense and Simons, 1999).
- MTrPs show greater density of immunoreactivity to substance P (a marker for peripheral sensitization) compared with normal muscle (De Stefano et al., 2000).
- The precise location of MTrPs can be identified reliably by two examiners independently (Sciotti et al., 2001).
- Extracellular fluid surrounding an MTrP and collected by microdialysis (Shah et al., 2005) contains higher concentrations than normal of several known substances that sensitize high-threshold nerve fibres in muscle. These include protons (H +), bradykinin, calcitonin gene-related peptide, substance P, tumour-necrosis factor-α, interleukin 1-β, serotonin and noradrenaline.

Many practitioners only discover MTrPs when they learn acupuncture; some describe it as a revelation in their medical practice, especially in primary care, as they are now able to diagnose and treat many patients who were previously classified rather unsatisfactorily as 'functional', and perhaps dismissed as impossible to diagnose or treat.

Although MTrPs were described by Travell and Simons within the context of conventional medicine, they do seem to correlate rather well with aspects of traditional Chinese acupuncture. Common trigger points are often situated at known acupuncture points, and one landmark study found 100% correlation between MTrPs and acupuncture points (Melzack et al., 1977). Traditional acupuncturists have been using *ah shi* points for many years. An *ah shi* point is one which, when pressed, causes the patient involuntarily to shout out *ah shi*, which means 'Oh yes!' ('That is my pain' or 'That is unusually tender'). In addition, many of the traditional acupuncture meridians in part appear to map out patterns of referred pain from trigger points.

MTrPs are perhaps an example of how the best of the complementary and conventional approaches can be integrated; a significant step forward in patient care.

Definition

Travell and Simons defined an MTrP as a 'hyperirritable locus within a taut band of skeletal muscle, located in the muscle tissue or its associated fascia' (Travell and Simons, 1983).

An MTrP is a hyperirritable locus within a taut band of skeletal muscle.

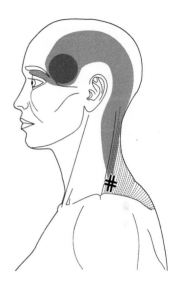

Figure 6.1   Myofascial trigger point in upper fibres of trapezius, referring pain mainly to the neck and temporal region.

The essential clinical features of an MTrP are:
- a taut band that can be palpated inside the belly of the muscle,
- part of the taut band is very tender,
- pressing that tender spot causes pain that the patient recognizes,
- movement of the joint that stretches the MTrP may be restricted by pain.

Pressure on an MTrP replicates the patient's pain when pressed.

An MTrP may be *active* and cause stiffness and pain or *latent* and cause stiffness without pain. An active MTrP may be inactivated by treatment, and a latent MTrP may be activated by a number of precipitating factors, which are described in Mechanisms.

MTrPs tend to occur in rather constant positions within muscles, for example, the anterior border of the upper fibres of trapezius (Fig. 6.1). Our diagrams mark the trigger point with cross-hatches (with the long strokes in the direction of the fibres) and the location of pain either in colour or with cross-hatching.

Many points in the body are tender; only MTrPs have all the characteristic features listed previously.

Incidence

MTrPs are common, and most people develop one or more during their lifetime. Physicians who are experienced in identifying trigger points can find at least one MTrP in about half of healthy, symptom-free young service personnel (Sola et al., 1955). In one study in primary care, MTrPs were found in 30% of patients consulting for pain (Skootsky et al., 1989). However, in reality they are not likely to be the *primary* cause of pain as frequently as this in civilian populations.

Aetiology

MTrPs may be caused by muscle injury or strain, but they may also occur secondary to other painful conditions. A strain that causes an MTrP in one patient may not bother a second patient – or even the same patient at another time, suggesting that there are other factors that make MTrPs more likely to develop. The same factors may prevent them from healing.

PRECIPITATING AND PERPETUATING FACTORS

Sometimes, the history of injury appears to be too trivial to have produced an MTrP, in which case the muscles may have been in a particularly vulnerable state. This can happen for a variety of reasons:

- emotional: stress and anxiety, excitement
- physical: exhaustion, poor muscle fitness from lack of exercise or exposure to cold
- metabolic: poor nutritional status, low vitamin levels, hypothyroidism or chronic infection.

These factors that precipitate an MTrP also perpetuate it and will also interfere with the response to treatment. They may need to be corrected before treatment can be successful and lasting.

Emotional, physical or metabolic factors can perpetuate an MTrP.

MYOFASCIAL TRIGGER POINTS FROM ACUTE OR CHRONIC MUSCLE STRAIN

Trigger points may arise rapidly in the few days following an acute strain of the muscle, or they may arise insidiously following chronic strain.

Most MTrPs are caused by muscle injury – acute or chronic.

The commonest acute strain occurs when the muscle is overloaded, for example, from lifting something too heavy or at an awkward angle. One muscle that is vulnerable to sudden overuse strain is pectoralis major (Fig. 6.2), most commonly in young men who lift heavy weights. Quadratus lumborum (Fig. 6.3), which is crucial in providing lateral support for the back, can easily be strained by lifting excessive weight with one hand. In these cases, the onset of pain is usually rapid.

Myofascial pain of gradual onset is likely to be caused by chronic, cumulative strain. This is common, for example, in the trapezius when many hours are spent working in poor posture. A postural abnormality, such as kyphosis or scoliosis, puts extra strain on the muscles of the trunk (e.g. quadratus lumborum) or neck (e.g. trapezius). Constant mental tension can also produce prolonged muscle contraction; for example, tightly hunched shoulders may cause MTrPs to develop in the neck muscles, particularly the trapezius.

Very occasionally, direct injury to the muscle can give rise to an MTrP, for example, when it is compressed for a long period (e.g. sitting in a chair where the front edge compresses the hamstrings).

Because of the way MTrPs are caused by injury, they are often unilateral.

Primary MTrPs are usually unilateral.

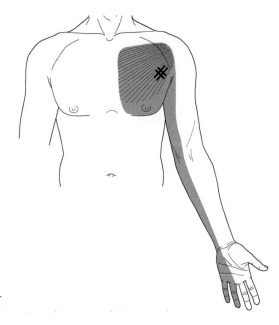

Figure 6.2 Myofascial trigger point in pectoralis major, referring pain to chest and arm.

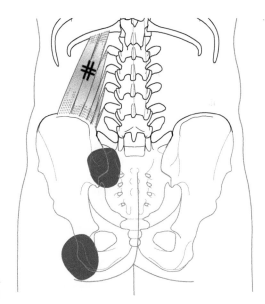

Figure 6.3 Myofascial trigger point in quadratus lumborum, referring pain to sacrum and buttock.

OTHER CAUSES OF MYOFASCIAL TRIGGER POINTS

MTrPs can develop in painful conditions and then cause added problems for the patient. This is referred to as secondary myofascial pain. For example, arthritis of the hip is associated with MTrPs in the gluteal muscles, and MTrPs may develop in pectoralis major after myocardial infarction. This can lead to a confusing clinical picture as two diagnoses can be implicated for one set of symptoms. It is important to diagnose the original condition and give definitive treatment, but it may also be helpful to treat the MTrPs.

There is a strong relationship between the abdominal viscera and the muscles of the abdominal wall, via the nervous system (see Chapter 8). MTrPs can develop in the abdominal muscle wall after an acute condition, such as gastroenteritis.

The diagnosis of an MTrP is not complete until an underlying cause is identified (whether injury or other condition).

Whenever pain occurs, including serious conditions such as cancer, an MTrP may also occur and confuse the diagnosis. Therefore we cannot overemphasize the importance of making a conventional diagnosis.

Mechanisms

An MTrP is best regarded as a pathophysiological disorder rather than a purely pathological one, so 'mechanism' is a more appropriate term than 'pathology'. An MTrP feels distinctly hard, and it is rather surprising that microscopy of biopsy specimens shows no corresponding major pathology. Most research on the mechanisms of MTrPs has concentrated on the muscle fibres rather than the overlying fascia, and that is the approach that we reflect here.

Electrical activity has been detected from electromyography (EMG) needles placed within 1 mm of an MTrP (Hubbard and Berkoff, 1993). This activity arises in muscle end plates and is called 'miniature end plate potentials' (MEPPs). It shows the effect of the release of packets of acetylcholine (ACh) in an excessive fashion. It is this persistent release of ACh that is the basic marker of an MTrP. Mense and Simons (1999) have proposed a hypothesis (Fig. 6.4) in which trauma to the end plate sets off the following sequence:

- sustained release of ACh leading to prolonged depolarization
- calcium depletion
- disturbed membrane function disturbs depolarization wave over muscle cell wall
- local contracture of sarcomeres in the immediate vicinity of the end plates
- muscle shortening to form taut band (this should be distinguished from muscle spasm, which entails coordinated contraction of whole muscle belly)

Although this is still a hypothesis and not yet an established mechanism, one of the predictions that arise from it has been supported in further experimentation: there is an accumulation of nociceptive transmitters around an MTrP (Shah et al., 2005).

Clinical features

PRESENTING SYMPTOMS

Patients with active MTrPs usually present with a deep, dull, aching pain. More rarely, they present with associated stiffness or restriction of movement. Symptoms can vary greatly in severity – both between different patients and over time in the same patient – often for no obvious reason. In everyday activities we are unaware of normal muscle tension until nerve endings are sensitized within MTrPs, then we become aware of the tension, especially in postural muscle, and it seems unconnected with activity.

MTrP pain is usually deep and aching and fluctuates for no apparent reason.

Dysfunctional endplate region

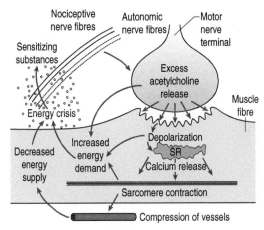

Figure 6.4   Integrated hypothesis of mechanism of myofascial trigger point. The primary dysfunction hypothesized here is an abnormal increase (by several orders of magnitude) in the production and release of acetylcholine packets from the motor nerve terminal under resting conditions. The greatly increased number of miniature end plate potentials (MEPPs) produces end plate noise and sustained depolarization of the postjunctional membrane of the muscle fibre. This sustained depolarization could cause a continuous release and inadequate uptake of calcium ions from local sarcoplasmic reticulum (SR) and produce sustained shortening (contracture) of sarcomeres. Each of these four highlighted changes would increase energy demand. The sustained muscle fibre shortening compresses local blood vessels, thereby reducing the nutrient and oxygen supplies that normally meet the energy demands of this region. The increased energy demand in the face of an impaired energy supply would produce a local energy crisis, which leads to release of sensitizing substances that could interact with autonomic and sensory (some nociceptive) nerves traversing that region. Subsequent release of neuroactive substances could, in turn, contribute to excessive acetylcholine release from the nerve terminal, completing what then becomes a self-sustaining vicious cycle. *(Reproduced with permission from Simons, D.G., Travell, J.G., Simons, L.S., 1999. Travell and Simons' Myofascial Pain and Dysfunction: The Trigger Point Manual, vol. 1. Upper Half of Body, second ed. Williams & Wilkins, Baltimore.)*

The pain is usually referred away from the MTrP, and the painful zone may not even include the MTrP itself. For example, the trapezius refers pain to the neck and head, and there may be little pain at the site of the MTrP. The pain referral pattern for each muscle is reasonably consistent, so an accurate description is important in identifying the MTrP.

The patterns are often reminiscent of the 'channels' of traditional Chinese acupuncture, and they may well be the same phenomenon (Hong, 2000). For example, the MTrP in the trapezius is at the location of GB21, and the pain referral zone is remarkably similar to the Gall Bladder channel as shown in Figure 6.5.

The pain pattern may reveal the location of the MTrP.

Patients with very active MTrPs show a characteristic clinical picture: the pain is deep, gripping and unremitting; the patient is restless, continually pressing deep and hard in the painful area or stretching the affected part to try to relieve the pain. Movement may ease the pain and patients may even walk the streets at night in an attempt to escape the pain. If the patient can get rest in bed, the pain may be set off again if the muscle is kept shortened. For example, a patient with an MTrP in the left pectoralis major who sleeps on their side with the left arm folded across the chest is likely to wake in pain from the shortened muscle. Patients might sit or lie in an unnatural

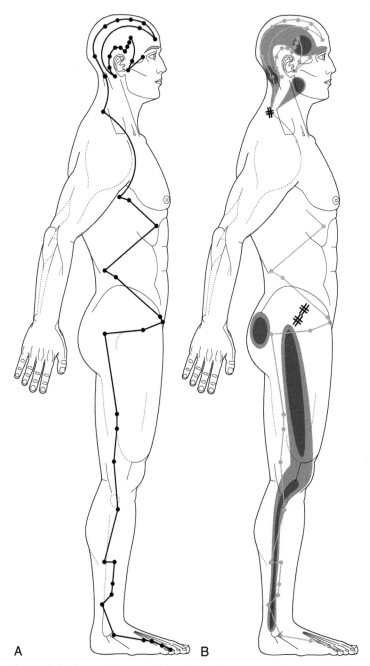

Figure 6.5 The correlation between trigger points and acupuncture points. (A) The trigger point in the upper fibres of trapezius is equivalent to the classical point GB21 and refers pain around the neck and head in a way that is remarkably similar to the GB meridian. (B) The trigger points in gluteus minimus are close to GB29 and GB30 (allowing for variation due to the patient's position) and refer pain down the leg to the ankle, in a pattern which is very close to the classical description of the GB meridian.

posture to keep the muscle in a lengthened position – the 'position of ease'. Patients often try to relieve the pain with a hot shower or bath.

The pain from an acute MTrP may simulate a medical or surgical emergency.

Less active MTrPs produce a less dramatic clinical picture: the pain and stiffness seem similar in many ways to the picture of osteoarthritis, which often coexists. The pain is often deep and aching in nature, and the stiffness is worst after immobilization and eases with exercise.

HISTORY: DIRECT QUESTIONING

It is important to obtain a precise history of the injury in cases of sudden onset and details of physical activities at work in cases of insidious onset. Aggravating and relieving factors may help in establishing which muscle contains the MTrP. Pain due to MTrPs is often worse in cold weather, at times of stress and anxiety, and just before or during menstruation.

A few MTrPs have pathognomonic symptoms, such as superficial prickling sensations over the chin and face from MTrPs in the platysma. Interested practitioners can discover these with experience, as long as they keep an open mind about the cause of 'peculiar' symptoms and keep a copy of a detailed reference book close at hand, such as Travell and Simons' manual.

HISTORY: OTHER SYMPTOMS

Occasionally, autonomic symptoms dominate the clinical picture; for example, one MTrP in the sternomastoid muscle causes dizziness and disorientation as well as pain.

The shortening and swelling of some muscles lead to pressure on nearby nerves and produce symptoms of nerve entrapment. For example, an MTrP in the piriformis can compress the sciatic nerve as it passes through the greater sciatic foramen. The patient may complain not only of the pain in a typical referral pattern, but also of paraesthesiae and numbness in the leg, as shown in Figure 6.6. This combination of symptoms is easily confused with sciatica caused by nerve-root compression.

TRIGGER POINTS AND SPINAL PAIN

MTrPs commonly cause spinal pain or at least contribute to it. Low back pain may be produced by MTrPs in muscles of the various paravertebral groups (multifidi, longitudinal group, additional muscles such as quadratus lumborum) or the hip girdle, such as piriformis. Neck pain may be due to MTrPs in the neck muscles or in the shoulder girdle muscles, such as trapezius. Patients who have been told their x-ray films show 'degenerative change' may actually have pain that is due to MTrPs.

MTrPs may mimic other medical conditions.

Diagnosis

A convincing diagnosis of an MTrP can be made when the following features are found on history and examination:
- a history of pain that fluctuates for no good reason
- a taut band in the muscle
- an area of tenderness in the taut band

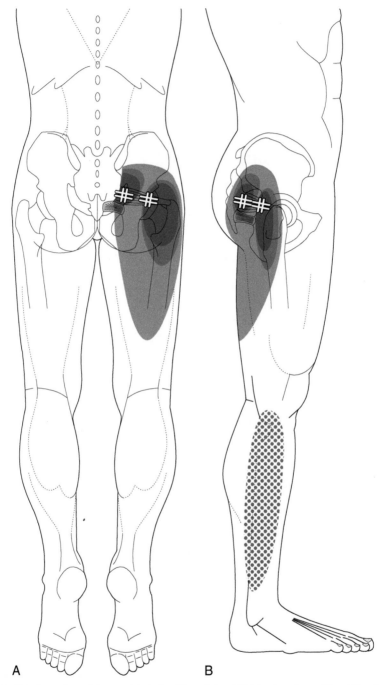

Figure 6.6   This figure shows trigger points in the (A) medial and (B) lateral sections of the piriformis muscle, which can lead to shortening of the muscle. This shortening compresses the sciatic nerve, causing paraesthesia in the lower leg. The important point to note is that paraesthesiae in the leg are not invariably caused by lesions to the nerve root.

- patient's pain reproduced by pressure on the tender area
- passive stretch of the involved muscle restricted by pain

Proper examination for MTrPs requires a good knowledge of anatomy, and many acupuncturists find they need to relearn the attachments and functions of muscle.

PALPATION

It is important to be able to identify an MTrP by palpation to make the diagnosis and needle it precisely. It is crucially important to draw the fingers *across* the muscle, at right angles to the fibres. Many clinicians are used to feeling through muscles to the structure below; this is one of the rare occasions when it is the muscle fibres themselves that are of interest.

Firstly, prepare and position the patient so that the muscle is:

- not tense – the patient has to be warm, relaxed and comfortable, with any affected limb well supported. This usually involves treating the patient lying down, with pillows for support;
- accessible – a limb might have to be placed in a particular position; for example, pectoralis major in the anterior axillary wall can only be examined fully with the arm abducted; quadratus lumborum can only be accessed with the patient lying on the opposite side, with the upper leg lowered right on to the couch to open the angle between the ribs and the iliac crest;
- the right length – if the fibres are fully stretched the taut band may not be palpable; if fully shortened the bulk of the muscle hides the MTrP. The appropriate length is achieved by moving the limb, for example, increasing or decreasing the abduction of the arm when examining pectoralis major.

Examine for MTrPs by drawing the fingers across the muscle fibres.

There are two techniques for palpation: flat or pincer (see Fig. 6.7). In both cases the fingers are drawn across the fibres. Flat palpation is suitable for most muscles, such as quadratus lumborum or the medial portion of pectoralis major. But if part of the muscle can be lifted off underlying structures – for example, the upper trapezius, the lateral portion of pectoralis major in the anterior axillary fold, or the teres major and latissimus dorsi in the posterior axillary fold – the examiner's fingers and thumb encircle the muscle and gently and systematically palpate it between the tip of a finger and the tip of the thumb. It does not take long to learn to recognize normal muscle

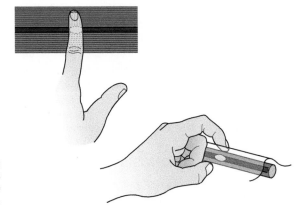

Figure 6.7 Diagrams showing flat palpation of myofascial trigger points and pincer palpation when the muscle belly can be encircled with the fingers.

fibre density and to identify the thicker, harder 'taut band', like a rope running the length of the muscle.

Having identified the band, then examine it gently for a tender spot, which is the MTrP itself, usually at about the midpoint. Finally, press on the tender spot for about 5 seconds and ask the patient what he or she feels. The best response is: 'That's my pain' (i.e. pain recognition). Be careful not to hint that that is the response you want, as some patients will be eager to please you or may not realize that there is an alternative option (i.e. that it is a different pain in the same place as their own pain). The patient's pain is more likely to be reproduced by needling because this applies pressure that is greater than that of the fingertip and concentrated in the muscle.

Forceful examination can aggravate MTrPs.

TWITCH RESPONSE

Trigger points may show another clinical sign on palpation – the twitch response – but remember that this may be painful and is not necessary for diagnosis. It is produced by 'snapping' palpation, which involves a firmer pull or tweak across the fibres, rather like twanging a guitar string in slow motion. It appears as a brief twitch under the skin, in line with the MTrP. It does not involve the whole muscle, like a tendon reflex, and should be distinguished from the effect of simply snapping the muscle border. Twitch responses should be generated during treatment with the needle, since they are regarded as a sign that treatment is likely to be effective.

A twitch response, with pain recognition, from needling is likely to indicate a favourable outcome.

DIFFICULTIES IN MYOFASCIAL TRIGGER POINT EXAMINATION

Palpation is not always straightforward. In deeper muscles, such as piriformis, the MTrP is not accessible. In these cases, a careful history is important, and examination for limitation of range of movement and weakness is necessary. In addition, compare the two sides. MTrPs are generally unilateral, at least in the early stages. Accurate palpation is difficult in patients who are obese.

MTrP pain is usually limited to one side (of the midline).

Patients rarely have a single MTrP; other nearby muscles are also likely to develop MTrPs. It is important to note that both the target area and the trigger point may be tender: only the MTrP has the taut band, tender nodule and pain recognition on pressure. When practitioners first start examining muscles, they often find difficulty in distinguishing between tender points (there are often many) and MTrPs (there are usually few). The key to success is to concentrate on developing the feel for a taut band. Diagnosis becomes easier with experience and practice, but sometimes it is simply not possible to be sure if a particular tender point is the origin of the pain. In this case it is entirely justifiable to treat the point speculatively, but carefully, as a 'therapeutic trial'.

Tenderness of the pain reference zone can be a distraction; the MTrP itself must be found.

DIFFERENTIAL DIAGNOSIS

Suspect an MTrP if the clinical picture suggests a musculoskeletal condition (i.e. is related to activity), but does not precisely match another clinical diagnosis. Anomalous symptoms that are

TABLE 6.1 ■ **Myofascial trigger points that develop secondary to medical conditions and produce a similar clinical picture**

Original condition	Persistent functional diagnosis	Muscles typically involved	Somatovisceral symptoms
Myocardial infarction	Postinfarction pain	Pectoralis major	Chest pain
Oesophagitis	Chronic epigastric pain	Rectus abdominis	Epigastric burning pain, nausea, anorexia, vomiting
Gastroenteritis	Irritable bowel syndrome	Rectus abdominis, internal obliques and external obliques	Pain, diarrhoea, constipation, bloating
Cystitis	Chronic cystitis	Lower rectus abdominis	Lower abdominal pain and frequency of micturition
Dysmenorrhoea	Chronic pelvic pain	Lower rectus abdominis	Cramping lower abdominal and pelvic pain

often labelled 'atypical' or 'idiopathic' could be due to MTrPs, for example, atypical facial pain. Several conditions may give rise to MTrP pain that persists and may cause difficulty in diagnosing a chronic problem, as shown in Table 6.1.

INVESTIGATIONS

There are no investigations that can assist the diagnosis of MTrPs. Thermography has been suggested but subsequently rejected as unreliable. Ultrasound and MRI have not, up to now, revealed any diagnostic features. Electromyography may be diagnostic but is only relevant as a research tool. Blood tests are of no value, except that they may be useful to exclude hypothyroidism if this is clinically suspected, because it may cause resistance to treatment.

Treatment techniques

Needling is not the only way to treat MTrPs, but it is quick and effective. This section is not intended on its own to give enough information to guide treatment with needles; full details of needling techniques are given in Chapter 15. There are four general approaches to needling MTrPs:

1. Direct, deep needling, which means inserting the needle directly into the MTrP itself. This is swift and effective for acute MTrPs. The practitioner must know the local anatomy to avoid serious harm. Very often the MTrP is not located on the first thrust of the needle and repeated thrusts are needed, spreading in a fanlike pattern from the skin insertion point (called 'fanlike lift and thrust') (Fig. 15.2). Direct needling seems to have a local effect, but it is not clear precisely what that is. It may simply physically disrupt the dysfunctional unit (considering the size of the needle in relation to muscle fibres, Fig 6.8) and perhaps provoke local vasodilation, which assists tissue healing.

2. Superficial needling, which is simply inserting the needle into the tissues precisely over the site of the MTrP. When using this method, it is essential that all tender MTrPs are treated together in the treatment session and that treatment is repeated until they are no longer tender. The mechanism of this effect is unknown and not based on obvious anatomical connections, since the overlying skin usually has different innervation from the MTrP. It is very acceptable to patients and unlikely to cause reactions. It is particularly useful for treating MTrPs situated in an anatomical area where deep needling carries excess risk, for example, in the anterior neck or just medial to the scapula.

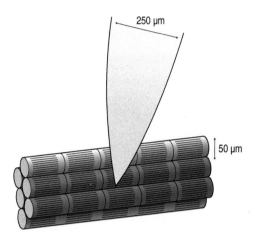

Figure 6.8 Tip of acupuncture needle in relation to skeletal muscle fibres, drawn to scale.

3. Needling local classical Chinese acupuncture points might have some effect on MTrPs, but the evidence is unclear.

4. Electroacupuncture (see Chapter 15) is mainly used to treat chronic MTrPs. Insert one needle into the MTrP, the other a few centimetres away along the MTrP band.

However, in treating chronic myofascial pain in relatively insensitive and acupuncture unresponsive patients, more vigorous techniques with multiple muscle twitches may both be acceptable and carry the most benefit.

After needling MTrPs, ask the patient to move the affected part through its full range of movement, slowly and deliberately, to achieve a gentle stretch. This helps to inactivate the MTrP and re-educate both the muscle and its owner that the muscle shortening has been abolished and the range of movement is normal. At the same time, warn patients not to overload the muscle.

After needling, stretch the muscle slowly – but do not overload it.

Patients should also be warned that they may feel soreness in the muscle for a few hours after treatment and can use a hot-water bottle, bath, shower or their usual analgesic medication for relief. Simple analgesics seem more effective than non-steroidal anti-inflammatory drugs.

These recommendations on needling are based on clinical experience, since there is little definitive research on treatment techniques. Some practitioners, particularly in the United States, inject MTrPs with local anaesthetic, saline, steroid solution or botulinum toxin, but a systematic review found none of these was superior to dry needling (Tough et al., 2009). Botulinum toxin has a theoretical advantage since it blocks release of acetylcholine and thus may 'switch off' the pathophysiological mechanism of the MTrP at its source, but early studies have been disappointing. Other physical therapies that are likely to work for MTrPs include deep massage and stretches of various sorts.

Prognosis

MTrPs of recent onset, limited to a single muscle and not overly active, may respond very swiftly to needling, possibly even to a single treatment. However, when MTrPs have developed in several muscles in a group and have been present for more than about 6 months, treatment needs to be repeated weekly for several weeks, and patients may need to work hard at active stretching exercises between treatments to reinforce the effect of needling. Also, bad postural habits should be corrected, as they perpetuate the problem. Chronic MTrPs may not dissipate permanently but may revert to being latent MTrPs.

A patient can reduce the likelihood of reactivating latent MTrPs by continuing a daily stretching routine, keeping the muscle warm, and avoiding overload, which includes correcting underlying ergonomic or postural stresses.

It is interesting to note that some patients who have had successful MTrP therapy feel a major improvement in their general well-being. The physical limitation, pain, and sleep disturbance caused by the MTrP had adverse effects on their lives in ways that they had not recognized until they were treated. This fact may contribute to the improvement in well-being that is frequently reported as a general benefit after acupuncture treatment.

Summary

MTrPs arise when a muscle or its associated fascia fail to heal after injury, and MTrPs should be distinguished from other tender points. The mechanism of MTrPs probably involves sustained release of acetylcholine at the muscle end plate and chronic contraction of adjacent sarcomeres. They present with pain, and the pain pattern often indicates where the MTrP lies. MTrPs are diagnosed by a palpable taut band with a tender point and patient recognition of pain. Precise needling of the MTrP followed by putting the muscle through its full range of movement can often inactivate it. The prognosis is good if treated early and any perpetuating factors can be removed.

Further reading

Baldry, P.E., 2005. Acupuncture, Trigger Points and Musculoskeletal Pain, third ed. Elsevier, Edinburgh.
   This text provides a thorough explanation of the most common myofascial trigger points encountered in practice. The author recommends treatment by superficial needling.
Simons, D.G., Travell, J.G., Simons, L.S., 1999. The Trigger Point Manual, second ed. Williams & Wilkins, Baltimore.
   This two-volume manual is expensive but regarded as the canon of myofascial trigger point pain. Full of terrific detail and wonderful anatomical diagrams to serve as a handbook for a lifetime of practice.

Segmental effects I: analgesia

Introduction

This chapter explains how acupuncture brings pain relief to the area around the needle according to the *gate control* theory of pain, in addition to the local effects that were discussed in Chapter 5.

The important concept of *segmental treatment* is introduced here. This has its origins in the segmental organization of the body, and to understand this we need to look briefly at foetal development. The concept of segmental innervation as applied to *dermatomes* is widely known and used, for example, in testing for damage to sensory nerves. Here the concept is extended to sclerotomes (sensory), viscerotomes (autonomic) and myotomes (both sensory and motor).

During the first weeks of growth, the human foetus is clearly organized in a segmental manner. But as it develops, many of the organs and other structures migrate. They drag their nerve supply with them, always maintaining their original innervation. Tissues from different layers, such as skin, muscle and viscera, may migrate in different directions. Therefore in the adult, tissues that are anatomically far apart may be innervated by the same spinal segment.

Just as a *dermatome* indicates the area of skin supplied by a single spinal segment, so also the muscles, internal organs and periosteum can be organized by their segmental level, as shown in Table 7.1 and the example in Figure 7.1.

At each segmental level, sensory information from that segment's dermatome, myotome, sclerotome and viscerotome *converges* in the dorsal horn. This information can change the way nociceptive information is handled, for example, 'closing the gate' to pain. The gate is controlled both directly by the incoming fibres (we are particularly interested in type III fibres from ergoreceptors, of course) and indirectly by descending control from a midbrain centre.

The afferent information also changes the activity of the autonomic reflex operating within the segment, which will be discussed in the next chapter.

Thus needles inserted close to a painful area can relieve the pain by 'closing the gate' in the dorsal horn.

Throughout this chapter, we discuss a 'segment' as if it receives all the input from the receptors in its receptive field and acts in isolation from its neighbours. Yet neither of these statements is strictly true. Sensory nerves usually ascend a segment or two as they enter the cord, and they have an input into several adjacent segments. Similarly, adjacent segments are known to intercommunicate, and their outputs tend to be similar.

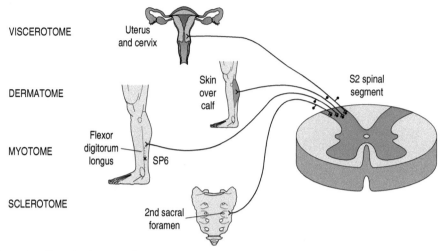

Figure 7.1 Example of segmental treatment approach: convergence of afferent information at S2 from uterus (viscerotome), skin over calf (dermatome), flexor digitorum longus (myotome, needled at SP6) and periosteum close to second sacral foramen (sclerotome, though this is rarely used in practice).

Case History

A physical therapist has been asked to help an 82-year old lady with chronic, though moderate, osteoarthritis (OA) of her knees. A conservative approach is appropriate as her pain and imaging of the knee joints is not sufficient to warrant knee replacement surgery, and in addition she also is overweight and has mild heart failure.

The therapist knows that getting the patient to walk more and exercise her knees is essential for long-term benefit, but the patient is reluctant because of the pain.

So the therapist gives her a few sessions of acupuncture. The first time, she simply inserts four needles deep into some acupuncture points in the muscles above and below the knee. On the patient's return the following week, she reports little benefit, so this time the therapist uses the same needle placement but adds electrical stimulation for 20 minutes. After two further weekly treatments, the patient reports relief, starts mobilizing again and gets out of the house.

TABLE 7.1 ▣ Terminology of '-tomes' and their relevance to acupuncture

Tissue	-tome name	Relevance
Skin	Dermatome	Dermatome charts are well known
Muscle	Myotome	Commonly used in acupuncture to modulate particular spinal segments (many examples are provided in Chapter 19)
Organ	Viscerotome	Discussed in the next chapter, for autonomic control
Periosteum, bone	Sclerotome	Used in periosteal pecking (examples provided in Chapter 19)

Another point to note is that the skin and the underlying muscles may be innervated by different segments, so a single needle may stimulate more than one segment.

The advantage to the acupuncturist concerning all this intercommunication and overlapping is this: although it is best to place the needle in the precisely correct segment (Lundeberg et al., 1989), some effect will be seen from needling an adjacent segment.

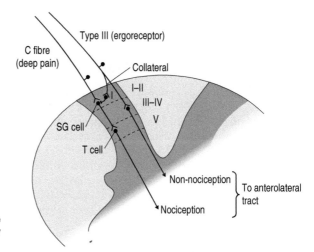

Figure 7.2 Diagram showing the principles of the gate control theory within the dorsal horn.

The overlap between segments also brings a disadvantage for clinical research, making it difficult or impossible to find a 'placebo' point for clinical trials. A placebo point has to be realistic to the patient – and therefore somewhere reasonably close to the source of pain – but must have no effect on the pain location. This difficulty is the likely cause of many 'false negative' clinical trials (see Chapter 12).

Mechanisms

We discuss here how the nociceptive pathway is inhibited by gate control, both directly by the afferent nerve and indirectly by descending inhibition.

GATE CONTROL THEORY OF PAIN

The gate control theory of Melzack and Wall (Melzack & Wall, 1965) provides a comprehensive, early explanation of the segmental analgesic effects of acupuncture, illustrated in Fig. 7.2.

Consider our patient with chronic knee pain from osteoarthritis. The noxious stimuli causing her pain arise in the pain-sensitive areas of the knee joint – probably the synovium, attachments of the joint capsule, periosteum and possibly also the subchondral bone. The nociceptive signals travel in the small unmyelinated C fibres into the dorsal horn, mainly at the levels L3/L4, L4/5 and L5/S1. The C fibres terminate mainly at the substantia gelatinosa (lamina II), activating a short pathway that normally stimulates the (transmission) neuron in lamina V. The nociceptive signal continues up the ascending, anterolateral tract. This projects mainly to the thalamus and on to conscious awareness of pain in the cortex, but a minority of the ascending fibres terminate at the brainstem and activate either the *reticular system* projecting to the limbic system or the *periaqueductal grey* (PAG), which is the origin of descending inhibition (DI).

To treat the pain, acupuncture points are chosen in the dermatome or myotome (more rarely, the sclerotome) of the segments that innervate the knee, L3 to S1.

Needles inserted into skin or connective tissue will stimulate Aβ fibres; those inserted into muscle will activate ergoreceptors, generating signals in type III fibres. The main axon of both types of fibre terminates in laminae III/IV and projects up the anterolateral tract. But these fibres also have a collateral fibre which closes the gate (or inhibits the nociceptive pathway), probably in two ways: (1) by releasing enkephalin, which directly inhibits the transmission cell; and (2) by stimulating inhibitory interneurons, which inhibit the transmission cell indirectly. In this way, the nociceptive pathway is intercepted in the spinal cord.

DESCENDING INHIBITION: THE 'LONG LOOP'

The gate can also be closed by *descending inhibition* (DI), descending from the periaqueductal grey (PAG). An example of the effect of DI can be seen when an injury is ignored while the person's attention is distracted. In this chapter we are not talking about activating DI by distraction but rather by type III fibres and the anterolateral tracts. These release β-endorphin in the midbrain, activating DI.

The PAG is organiszed in a somatotopic manner. Therefore fibres from each segment activate the part of the DI system that sends descending information back directly to that segment, an arrangement called 'long loop'. This long loop reflex is based on considerable laboratory evidence in animals and some in humans, and it has been shown that stimulation must be maintained for at least 10 minutes to activate DI.

The ways in which DI influences the nociceptive pathway include release of serotonin, which activates the (inhibitory) interneurons in the dorsal horn, and release of noradrenaline.

It is debated how much the direct spinal mechanisms and DI each contribute to acupuncture's effect. The precise workings of the dorsal horn are not yet sufficiently well understood to be exactly sure. In practice it makes little difference: any treatment that stimulates type III fibres (and their important collaterals) will also stimulate DI. The therapist should be aware of both mechanisms.

Clinical application

Segmental analgesia can be achieved with acupuncture by stimulating nerves in the same dermatome, myotome or sclerotome as the segment of origin of the pain. Our case study involves the knee, which is innervated by the femoral and sciatic nerves, so the relevant spinal segments are L2-5 and usually S1. As a general rule, selecting points around a joint will almost inevitably affect the relevant segments for the joint.

To find the *dermatomes* supplied by L2-5 segments, consult the dermatome diagram at the back of this book (Fig. 19.14). In general, the relevant dermatome lies over the painful area, but there are important exceptions, such as over the spinal column. Choose any known acupuncture points in that dermatome, maybe using examples given in Table 19.3.

In our case, the physiotherapist used her knowledge of *myotomes*. She placed needles in two acupuncture points: SP10 (Spleen 10) above the knee, needling vastus medialis (innervated by L2–4), and ST36 (Stomach 36) just below the knee, needling tibialis anterior (innervated by L4–5).

When treating joint pain, it is easier to be sure of the myotome than the dermatome because of a simple general rule: joints are innervated by the same segments that supply the muscles that act on them. So work out which muscles are acting on the joint and needle them, preferably in recognized acupuncture points.

For other structures, it may sometimes be necessary to look up the innervation in an anatomy book or website.

A segmental effect on a joint can be activated by needling any muscle that acts on the joint.

To apply a *sclerotome* approach, look up the relevant sclerotome in Table 19.3. Remember that the technique for needling sclerotomes, so-called 'periosteal pecking', is different from needling skin or muscle, as described in Chapter 15.

To judge the strength of treatment needed, remember that needling of subcutaneous tissues has a relatively weak effect compared with needling muscle (Ceccherelli et al., 2001). Chronic conditions such as osteoarthritis, at least in patients who show a typical response, will need several subcutaneous needles and considerable stimulation to gain a useful effect (although a few patients are highly responsive, including many with cancer). Stimulating muscles is likely to be more effective, so fewer needles may be sufficient.

In our case study, manual needling of four needles had no effect, so subsequent treatment was reinforced. One option is to increase the number of needles, but it was decided to increase the strength of stimulation by using EA. Experience shows that EA is often needed for good pain relief in chronic knee OA.

A further option for reinforcing treatment would be to add more needles in the adjacent segments, which can be effective because of the overlap between segments. In our case, one might place the patient into the lateral position and add the point BL40 in the popliteal crease. This could be particularly appropriate if the knee pain was referred to the back of the knee.

Needles need to be retained long enough to release enkephalin from the intermediate cells, at least 10 minutes.

Acupuncture analgesia can have knock-on effects that may lead to some improvement in the condition, not just pain relief. In this case the analgesia may reverse any increased muscle tone, hence encouraging mobilization, which in turn improves blood flow and healing.

The analgesia gradually wears off over several days but can be reinforced by repeating the acupuncture, and the benefits accumulate over a course of treatment. In this way, even chronic pain can respond to acupuncture.

Segmental analgesia may reduce any increased muscle tone, improving mobility and pain relief.

Summary

Acupuncture needles affect the functioning of the dorsal horn of the spinal segment, both directly through the afferent nerve and by a long loop involving the brainstem. The effect is mainly inhibition through release of various neuromodulators, known as 'gate control'. These can inhibit the passage of nociceptive signals through the dorsal horn. This effect can be achieved by stimulating dermatome, myotome or sclerotome.

Further reading

Campbell, A., 2001. Beyond Points and Meridians. Butterworth Heinemann, Oxford.
  A radical book that succeeds in demystifying acupuncture, describing a treatment approach based on identifiable treatment areas.
Hayhoe, S., 2016. Acupuncture for chronic pain. In: Filshie, J., White, A., Cummings, M. (Eds.), Medical Acupuncture: A Western Scientific Approach, second ed. Elsevier, Edinburgh, pp 315–344.
  A summary of evidence and clinical approach for acupuncture treatment of conditions seen in a typical pain clinic.

Segmental effects II: autonomic modulation

Introduction

This chapter describes how to address certain medical conditions by using a segmental approach to modulate the body's autonomic activity. It refers principally therefore to the *visceral* effects of acupuncture.

The autonomic system generates a continuous (though variable) outflow or *tone* that achieves homoeostasis by controlling the function of bodily organs. The tone is constantly adjusted according to the individual's emotional and physical state and as a reflex response to information from the viscera themselves. The tone is a balance between sympathetic outflow, which prepares the body for 'fright, fight or flight', and parasympathetic outflow, which dominates everyday, regular, vegetative functions, sometimes referred to as 'rest and digest'.

The sympathetic outflow is powered by neurons in the lateral horns of the spinal column in the thoracic and lumbar regions; the parasympathetic by neurons in the vagal nucleus and lateral horns in the sacral spinal cord. These neurons are under both local and central (descending) control. This chapter principally discusses the spinal reflex, and central control is covered in Chapter 10. Individual organs differ regarding which type of control dominates: the bladder and bowel are largely controlled by spinal reflex, whereas the heart and circulation are under supraspinal (brainstem) control.

The visceral disturbances most commonly treated by acupuncture involve the gastrointestinal (GI) tract and the bladder. In both cases, autonomic disturbances are generally indicated by pain and by dysfunction. Irritable bowel syndrome is typified by the case history (see following page). A similar disturbance of bladder leads to 'irritable bladder' with urgency, bladder discomfort, urinary frequency, nocturia and passing small amounts of urine.

Stimulation of nociceptive nerves in the bowel or bladder activates spinal reflexes that increase the contraction of smooth muscle in the organ wall and stimulate mucosal secretion. Acupuncture impedes the pathway for visceral nociception in the same way as it inhibits somatic nociception, reducing the response of the dorsal horn neurons. In this way, it inhibits the autonomic reflex involving the lateral horn neuron to any nociceptive information arriving there from the viscera. So acupuncture can inhibit nociceptive stimuli from visceral structures such as the gut, bladder and uterus. An example is shown in Figure 8.1.

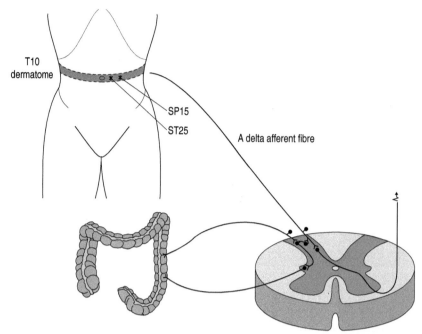

Figure 8.1 Subcutaneous needling of acupuncture points ST25 and SP15 in the appropriate dermatome inhibits the autonomic reflex involving the small intestine at segmental level T10. The collateral of the A delta fibre releases GABA and enkephalin in lamina II, inhibiting the autonomic pathway. Similar effects can be seen with stimulating type III fibres by needling underlying abdominal muscle, such as rectus abdominis, in the appropriate myotome.

Case History

A 30-year-old female office worker complained of a recurrence of her abdominal pain and urgency of bowel action, with alternating constipation and diarrhoea. The condition has been present for several years and fluctuates in severity, probably in association with periods of stress.

   She received six sessions of acupuncture in which needles were inserted at tender points over the abdomen. Needles were inserted into the deep subcutaneous layer or outer part of the underlying muscle and left for 10 minutes. The number of abdominal points used increased from just four to eight, with gentle manual stimulation, over the treatment course. In addition, a point on the foot (LR3) was needled bilaterally from the third treatment onwards: though this point is not in a myotome that is relevant to the bowel, it is often used to reinforce the effect of purely local needling.

   Her symptoms gradually resolved, leaving her more comfortable and with almost normal bowel function. She was told the condition may relapse in which case the acupuncture should be effective again.

   Acupuncture can also influence the supraspinal autonomic centre, modulating sympathetic outflow, as discussed in Chapter 10.

Mechanisms

The afferent arms of visceral nociception and dysfunction were introduced in Chapter 3. In brief, distension of the bowel activates mechanoreceptors, and abnormal (e.g. inflammatory) chemicals activate chemoreceptors. Afferent signals travel in thinly myelinated Aδ fibres and unmyelinated C fibres that follow the same route as the efferent nerves of the autonomic system (though in the opposite direction, naturally). Thus those travelling with sympathetic nerves enter the thoracic and lumbar spinal cord, and those travelling with parasympathetic nerves enter the vagal nucleus in the medulla and the sacral spinal cord.

Some autonomic afferents terminate in the substantia gelatinosa of the dorsal horn, then project to the lateral horn, where the cell bodies of the autonomic *efferents* are situated. In the case of the vagal nerve, the equivalent cell bodies are in the vagal nucleus of the medulla. Other afferent fibres pass into the dorsal columns and terminate in the brainstem, to impact on the autonomic centre, and also project to the limbic system (for the emotional responses) as well as the cortex (for awareness of the ache).

ROLE OF ACUPUNCTURE

Acupuncture has two effects on the autonomic nervous system – short term and long term – which are often in opposite directions. The moment needles are inserted, they may evoke a strong sympathetic reflex in the segment. This can be useful clinically; for example, in acute attacks of hay fever, acupuncture points close to the nose can dramatically open the nasal airway by vaso-constricting the nasal mucosa, reducing oedema and inhibiting mucous secretions. The response seems to be related to the strength of stimulation and can continue for some time after treatment.

If acupuncture stimulation is continued for at least 10 minutes, it can induce an inhibition of sympathetic outflow, which can persist well beyond the duration of needling. This effect appears to include both spinal reflex and supraspinal centres. There is clear laboratory evidence for inhibition of the spinal reflex to bladder, and clinical evidence supports this effect.

CONVERGENCE IN THE DORSAL HORN

Each dorsal horn receives afferents from the viscera (such as the bowel) and from somatic structures (the skin and muscles of the abdominal wall). These two afferent pathways *converge* into a single pathway at the dorsal horn, and the brain receives one type of signal, whether somatic or visceral in origin. Therefore pain from an abdominal organ is perceived as arising in the abdominal wall muscles that have the same segmental innervation. This is known as the 'viscerosomatic reflex'. Acupuncturists are exploiting this reflex when they use a segmental approach.

Afferent nerves from muscle and organ converge in the dorsal horn.

Clinical application

Acupuncture, given at the appropriate segmental site with the correct stimulation, can modulate the autonomic reflex to reduce pain and dysfunction. The segmental approach is relevant for bladder and bowel problems, whereas for modulating activity of heart and circulation, central control has to be targeted (see Chapter 10).

Acupuncture may treat the symptoms but will not change the underlying pathology. So it is important to know the diagnosis for the correct overall management of the patient.

In choosing a suitable point at which to treat a target organ, first identify at what segmental level the organ is represented (viscerotome) using Table 8.1 (or Table 19.2). Then choose an acupuncture point in the appropriate dermatome or myotome from Table 19.3.

A *dermatomal* approach is commonly used for GI or GU (genitourinary) problems and simply involves needling superficially at the site of pain or discomfort or at the suprapubic region for

TABLE 8.1 ■ Spinal segmental levels of autonomic innervation of the viscera

Viscera	Sympathetic	Parasympathetic
Heart	T1 to T5	
Lung and bronchi	T2 to T4	
Oesophagus (caudal part)	T5 to T6	vagus
Stomach	T6 to T10	
Small intestine	T9 to T10	
Large intestine to splenic flexure	T11 to L1	
Large intestine, splenic flexure to rectum	L1 to L2	S2 to S4
Liver and gallbladder	T7 to T9	Vagus
Testis and ovary	T10 to T12	Nil
Urinary bladder	T11 to T12	S2 to S4
Uterus	T12 to L1	S2 to S4

TABLE 8.2 ■ Commonly used acupuncture points in the leg and their innervation

Muscle	Acupuncture point	Myotome
Tibialis anterior	ST36	L4/5 (S1)
First dorsal interosseus (between hallux and second toe)	LR3	S2/S3
Flexor digitorum longus	SP6	S1/S2

painless bladder problems. Remember that the skin at the front of body has denser innervation than that of the posterior surface, so it probably has greater autonomic effects. Figure 16.15 shows that there are midline points at every level and rows of points over the centre and outer border of the rectus abdominis. Four points could be used at the first session, increasing subsequently if necessary. Needles can be inserted subcutaneously and left for 10–20 minutes.

With a *myotomal* approach, there are three groups of muscles you can use:

1. Muscles of the abdominal wall: the choice here is straightforward. Treat at the site of referred pain, because this must be the appropriate segment. This also applies in the thorax: treat the muscles where the pain is felt (though be very aware of the risk to the pleura, see Chapter 16).
2. Muscles in the paraspinal region: the choice here needs a little more thought. Treat paraspinal muscles at *approximately* the same level as the relevant spinous process. In practice, the longitudinal paraspinal muscles migrate some distance caudally during foetal development. But the short multifidi close to the vertebral column do not, so they can be relied on to be situated at their level of origin. The relevant point descriptions in Chapter 19 provide information on innervation of the muscles underlying the points you are likely to use.
3. Muscles in the lower limbs: the choice here needs a little more information. The myotomes of the peripheral acupuncture points cannot be guessed or calculated – we need to know the nerve supply of the underlying muscle. Table 8.2 gives the innervation of some muscles in the leg where common acupuncture points are situated. Do not worry if you do not already know these muscles. They will be like old friends by the time you have been practising acupuncture for a year or two. Again, the innervation of these muscles is presented in the relevant point descriptions in Chapter 19.

Treatment in the lower limbs should normally be bilateral. It is reasonable to expect stimulation of muscle points in the limbs to have greater general effects on the autonomic centre in the brainstem (see Chapter 10) than treatment to muscles of the abdominal wall. For example, to treat the uterus (S2/S4), we might choose to needle the flexor digitorum longus in the lower leg, at the point known as 'SP6' (S2).

It should be noted that segments that have sympathetic outflow can be accessed more easily than segments that have parasympathetic outflow. Since the vagus nerve is not accessible to acupuncturists (except, arguably, in the ear, see Chapter 17), the only accessible parasympathetics are at S2 to S4 levels. These are mainly used for moderating the contraction of detrusor muscle that empties the bladder. However, clinical experience suggests that stimulation of muscle points such as ST36 can have a marked effect on vagal tone.

STIMULATION

It is not really possible, in our present state of knowledge, to specify precisely how to use needle manipulation to increase or decrease the autonomic reflex at spinal level, except to say you should recall the general rule that painful needling will activate the sympathetic reflex temporarily. So it is probably best to increase the degree of stimulation until a response is seen (as when treating pain), regarding the effect of acupuncture to be normalizing the reflex response, whether increased or decreased.

Electroacupuncture can be used to increase the degree of stimulation, and a combination of low and intermediate frequency outputs (e.g. 2–4 Hz, 10–15 Hz) is probably best for regulating the autonomic system. Electrical stimulation of SP6 is virtually identical to a treatment known as 'posterior tibial nerve stimulation' (PTNS), which has been recommended by the National Institute for Health and Clinical Excellence (NICE) as a treatment for overactive bladder.

Abdominal organs can be influenced by treating points in the painful area of the abdomen.

While we suggest that intramuscular needling is the standard approach for achieving autonomic effects, other medical acupuncturists find superficial needling perfectly adequate for treating abdominal symptoms. They simply needle over the site of the pain.

Summary

Acupuncture can have useful effects on the autonomic reflexes that underlie some bladder and bowel disturbances, such as irritable bladder and irritable bowel. Incoming information from the organ is inhibited in the dorsal horn by acupuncture (non-nociceptive) stimulation. Dermatomal or myotomal approaches can be used.

General effects I: descending analgesia

Introduction

This chapter describes another of the body's inbuilt systems of self-regulation of pain and the ways that it can be activated by acupuncturists. *Descending inhibition* (DI) is a form of stimulation-produced analgesia and very much the workhorse of everyday acupuncture, for example, in treating osteoarthritis by placing needles around the joint.

We have already seen the effects of DI on the gate control of pain mechanism at the segmental level, in the dorsal horn – the 'long loop' reflex (Chapter 7). Descending inhibition supplements the effects of type III fibre stimulation in inhibiting the nociceptive pathway. This chapter discusses its central mechanisms and ways it might be activated.

We concentrate on descending inhibition of pain, but parallel descending systems can also enhance the perception of pain from a given nociceptive stimulus. These systems allow the brain to control the experience of pain – heightening awareness of pain when action needs to be taken to avoid harm, but reducing pain that does not represent danger. These systems are under a certain amount of conscious control, for example, using breathing or meditation techniques, as well as under subconscious influence, for example, being activated by psychological events such as distraction. They are influenced by personality and by situation – and, fortunately, by acupuncture.

It is not surprising therefore that acupuncture can recruit DI in ways other than the long loop reflex – that is, through effects on the *limbic system* and *default mode networks*, which will be described in more detail in Chapter 10. These are truly 'general' effects in that they affect the body overall and explain how acupuncture at sites that are some distance from the pain, such as auricular points or the well-known points in hands and feet, can generate a degree of analgesia. This can be useful for patients with widespread pain, such as fibromyalgia, or postoperatively.

Case History

A 54-year old-lady asked for acupuncture from her general practitioner for her trigeminal neuralgia, having tried several conventional therapies with no lasting success. She was currently in the middle of a severe attack. He asked her to lie on the couch for examination and needled LI4 unilaterally, gently manipulating the needle. Her neuralgia disappeared completely within a few minutes.

Subsequent acute episodes over several years continued to respond each time to needling of LI4, and after a while she learned to carry needles in her handbag and treat herself at the onset of pain.

After briefly introducing the pioneering research leading to the discovery that acupuncture releases opioid peptides, this chapter goes on to describe the mechanisms of DI and relevant neurophysiology of the opioid peptides before discussing suggested treatment regimens for activating DI.

EARLY RESEARCH INTO ACUPUNCTURE ANALGESIA

The first report of a proper objective assessment of acupuncture analgesia in humans was published in 1974 in a study on 60 Chinese medical students. They were given acupuncture at points in the hand (LI4) and knee (ST36) for 50 minutes, after which their threshold to painful electrical stimulation was found to be increased throughout the body – in the head, thorax, back, abdomen and leg (Research Group of Acupuncture Anaesthesia, 1974). Another seminal study showed that the analgesia involved a 'humoral factor' (Research Group of Acupuncture Anaesthesia, 1974). Cerebrospinal fluid (CSF) was drawn from a rabbit that was being given acupuncture and had demonstrated raised pain thresholds. The CSF was perfused into the cerebrospinal space of a second animal, which then developed a similar level of analgesia to the first. Clearly the CSF contained substances that were released by acupuncture, which we now recognize as neuromodulators.

Newer experimental methods have been developed to investigate the neurotransmitters and neuromodulators, and researchers throughout the world have been responsible for exploring the nature of the neurochemical response to acupuncture, but particularly Han in China (Han and Terenius, 1982) and Pomeranz in Canada (Pomeranz, 2001; Pomeranz and Chiu, 1976). More recently, our knowledge of these mechanisms has been extended enormously by the use of magnetic resonance imaging (MRI) techniques, particularly with functional MRI (Hui et al., 2005; Wu et al., 2002) and with positron emission tomography (PET) scanning (Harris et al., 2009; Pariente et al., 2005) .

Mechanisms

The DI system is based in the periaqueductal grey (PAG), a small group of cells in the midbrain (see Fig. 9.1). This is the nearest thing the body has to a 'pain control centre'. The PAG is the site at which the smallest dose of administered opioid drugs (e.g. morphine or heroin) can produce the most profound analgesic effect.

In the PAG's resting state, the descending inhibition systems are blocked by inhibitory neurons nearby. These inhibitory neurons can be 'switched off' by β-endorphin to activate the PAG inhibition (Zhao, 2008). This is a kind of triple negative: β-endorphin inhibits the neurons that inhibit the descending inhibitory system.

The active PAG neurons project to the nucleus raphe magnus (nRM), whose neurons project through the descending tract onto the dorsal horn of every segment in the spinal cord (Fig. 9.2). They release serotonin, which activates the inhibitory intermediate cells in the substantia nigra (lamina II) and in lamina V.

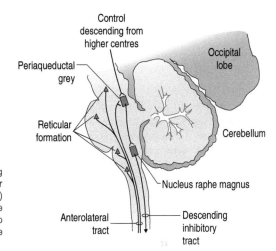

Figure 9.1 Diagram of brainstem showing anterolateral tract projecting to (1) reticular formation throughout brainstem and (2) periaqueductal grey (PAG). Also shown is the start of the descending inhibitory system to nucleus raphe magnus and onwards to the spinal cord.

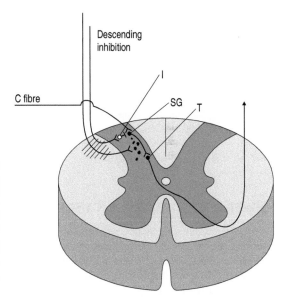

Figure 9.2 Diagram of the spinal cord showing descending inhibition: descending fibres release (1) serotonin, which activates inhibitory intermediate cells to release met-enkephalin, which inhibits nociceptive pathways and winds down the sensitivity within these pathways; and (2) noradrenaline, which diffuses through the dorsal horn and has inhibitory properties. Key: SG = substantia gelatinosa cell. T = transmission cell. I = intermediate cell (inhibitory).

The inhibitory neurons release enkephalin and probably GABA, which inhibit the transmission of nociception at slightly different positions. GABA causes presynaptic inhibition, that is, inhibiting the terminal of the afferent nerve, whereas enkephalin causes postsynaptic inhibition, affecting the second order neuron.

These descending effects are in addition to any segmental inhibition that is already activated at the segmental level through type III and Aβ neurons.

Descending inhibition is also provided by at least one other system that involves the locus coeruleus (not shown) and uses noradrenaline as the transmitter. Noradrenaline diffuses through the dorsal horn and has a direct inhibitory effect on the postsynaptic membrane of the neurons in laminae I, II and V, further reinforcing the effect of acupuncture on controlling nociception.

Descending inhibitory pain control inhibits the nociceptive pathway in the dorsal horn.

These particular actions of acupuncture are open to influence by pharmacological intervention. For example, tricyclic antidepressant drugs increase the release of both serotonin and noradrenaline in the central nervous system. There is some evidence that tricyclic antidepressants may be synergistic with acupuncture and increase its analgesic effect. Laboratory studies show that mice that are non-responsive to the analgesic effects of EA become responsive when they are given amitriptyline (Fais et al., 2012). Although selective serotonin reuptake inhibitors (SSRI) are not synergistic with EA, serotonin-noradrenaline reuptake inhibitors (SNRIs) increased the analgesic effect of EA in rats (Li et al., 2016).

Activation of descending inhibition

Descending inhibition can be activated in three ways, depending on where the stimulation is given (local or general) and what form it takes (standard or strong).

'LONG LOOP' ACTIVATION

This mechanism, central to acupuncture analgesia, was described in Chapter 7. In brief, acupuncture activates the anterolateral tract and a portion of these fibres pass directly to the PAG. The PAG is organized in a somatotopic manner: fibres from each spinal segment activate just the relevant portion of the PAG that inhibits that segment alone, hence the title 'long loop'.

This long loop reflex is supported by considerable laboratory evidence in animals and some in humans. Stimulation must be maintained for at least 10 minutes to activate DI.

It is worth noting that nociceptive C fibres follow the same afferent pathways in the spinal cord, so again a proportion of them will project to, and activate, the PAG as the body's inbuilt pain regulator.

GENERALIZED ACTIVATION THROUGH HIGHER CENTRES

In addition to receiving input from the anterolateral tract, the PAG is also under the control of the activity of higher centres in the brain. Several centres in the cortical and subcortical region can influence it, particularly the limbic system and functional networks such as the default mode network (DMN), described in Chapter 10. This provides a pathway by which (for example) distraction can temporarily inhibit pain of injury. The limbic system and the DMN are dysfunctional in patients with chronic pain, but acupuncture modulates them, normalizing their function.

ACTIVATION BY PAINFUL STIMULATION

The whole system of DI can also be activated by any painful stimulation. This process was originally known as 'diffuse noxious inhibitory control' (DNIC), but some now prefer the snappy term 'heterotopic noxious conditioning stimulus' (HNCS).

Traditionally, acupuncturists gave this painful stimulation at a single point in the leg ST37 to treat shoulder pain. Another example is strong stimulation of LR3, classically used to treat acute headache. There is no reason why the effect should be limited to shoulder pain and headache, but it does seem necessary to use a point at the far end of the body.

Another form of painful stimulation is periosteal pecking in which the needle is inserted deeply and repeatedly pushed against the periosteum with a tapping action.

Orthodox pain clinicians can often be heard dismissing acupuncture as simply a form of 'counterirritation' or DNIC, but since the majority of acupuncture treatments are comfortable and given near the site of pain, it seems unlikely that DNIC is the main mechanism in most circumstances.

Opioid peptides and acupuncture

All mechanisms of activating the PAG involve acupuncture's release of β-endorphin, the discovery of which first provided credibility for acupuncture in the scientific community. Four opioid peptides have now been identified, though their complete roles in pain perception are still not fully understood (Table 9.1). Each peptide is predominant in a different area of the CNS: *β-endorphin* is found in the brain and *enkephalin* in the spinal cord. Acupuncture causes both to be released. Dynorphin, in the spinal cord and brainstem, has variable effects depending on the circumstances. *Orphanin* (also known as 'endomorphin' or 'nociceptin') is widely distributed throughout the forebrain, midbrain and spinal cord and has a multitude of functions in nociception, other sensory functions and autonomic control (Han, 2004).

These opioid peptides are often referred to as neuro*modulators* rather than neuro*transmitters*, because they have a sustained effect and modify the activity of the target cell over a period of time.

Three types of opioid receptors have been identified, called 'μ' (mu), 'δ' (delta) and 'κ' (kappa). These are not matched exactly to the different peptides, and some of the peptides stimulate more than one receptor, as shown in Table 9.1.

β-endorphin plays an important role in acupuncture analgesia. In a piece of research that has become a landmark, acupuncture increased the concentrations of β-endorphin in the CSF of patients with pain, whereas control patients who did not receive acupuncture showed no changes (Clement-Jones et al., 1980). Subsequent studies have shown that the analgesic effect of acupuncture has a slow onset, reaches a peak after about 20 minutes, and then decays slowly after removing the needles (see Fig. 9.3). This time pattern is entirely consistent with the action of neuromodulator release.

The evidence that opioid peptides are involved in acupuncture has been reinforced by the discovery that some of the effects of acupuncture can be reversed by naloxone, both in the laboratory (Han and Terenius, 1982; Pomeranz and Chiu, 1976) and in clinical trials in patients with pain (Mayer et al., 1977). The discovery of specific antagonists to the different receptors has been crucially important in working out the roles of the different opioid peptides.

Acupuncture releases enkephalin in the spinal cord and β-endorphin in the brain.

TABLE 9.1 ■ **Comparison of the properties of the main opioid peptides in relation to acupuncture**

Peptide	Main site	Receptor	Blockage by naloxone	Relevant EA frequency (Hz)
β-endorphin	Midbrain, PAG	μ, δ	Low dose	Low (2–4)
Enkephalin	Dorsal horn of spinal cord	μ, δ	Low dose	Low (2–4)
Dynorphin	Brainstem and spinal cord	κ	High dose	High (50–100)
Orphanin	Widespread	μ	Unknown	Low (2–4)

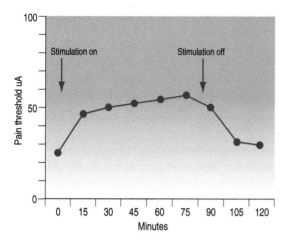

Figure 9.3 Graph indicating changes of dental pain threshold during electrical stimulation to needles in hands and cheeks, showing the delay in rise and fall of analgesia after onset and cessation of acupuncture (*Data from Anderson SA, Holmgren E, 1975. On acupuncture analgesia and the mechanism of pain. Am. J. Chin. Med. 3(4), 311–334. Reproduced with permission.*)

It is important to note that the previous discussion refers to the release of opioid peptides within the CSF. However, β-endorphin is also released from the pituitary directly into the bloodstream. This happens in response to several stimuli, not just acupuncture, and the precise role of this circulating β-endorphin in analgesia is not fully understood.

NATURAL OPIOID ANTAGONIST CHOLECYSTOKININ: ANXIETY

Cholecystokinin (CCK) is a naturally occurring antagonist of opioid peptides. It was named after being found to cause contraction of the gall bladder. Raised levels of CCK in the CNS are associated with an increased perception of pain; in addition, anxious patients have raised levels of CCK and, therefore, are likely to experience more pain.

To achieve the maximal benefit from opioid release, it is important to prepare patients for acupuncture in ways that reduce anxiety, such as avoiding rush, providing adequate explanation, and leaving opportunities for questions and discussion, as well as using touch, if appropriate. A relaxed patient will have lower levels of CCK and better results with acupuncture theoretically.

In addition, it is worth remembering that CCK is released by acupuncture in the laboratory when stimulation is prolonged for more than about 45 minutes. Acupuncture analgesia for postoperative pain control or for labour pain may need to be continued for more than 2 hours. Theoretically this continued stimulation could become counterproductive, though several studies have suggested that this is not a significant problem clinically.

OTHER GENERAL ANALGESIA MECHANISMS OF ACUPUNCTURE

It has been clear ever since the earliest days of neurophysiological research into acupuncture that the response to needling is complex, and that other transmitters, as well as opioids, are involved.

Oxytocin may have an important role in many of the effects of acupuncture, including analgesic, anxiolytic and sedative effects (Uvnas-Moberg et al., 1993; Yang et al., 2007). Oxytocin release is also generated by stroking, gentle massage and physical touch, particularly to the ventral surface of the body. The roles of oxytocin have been reviewed (Yang et al., 2013).

Analgesia can be produced by shock in some animals. The shock may include painful electrical stimulation in experiments that are supposed to be investigating (non-painful) acupuncture. The mechanism for this effect may be release of ACTH and β-endorphin from the pituitary into the

TABLE 9.2 ■ **Typical treatment to activate descending analgesia**

Point locations	Well-known points in and around the site of pain
Number of points used	Two or three, bilaterally
Depth of insertion	Into muscle
Needle stimulation	Manipulation of each needle, usually repeated; or high- and low-frequency EA
Sensation elicited	De qi, muscle contraction if using EA
Needle retention time	20 minutes

circulation. This can lead to some confusion in interpreting the findings of laboratory studies of electroacupuncture.

Clinical application

Descending inhibition can be activated by acupuncture to reinforce local and segmental analgesia.

Point selection is not likely to be critical. Descending inhibition of pain can probably be generated most effectively at the well-known major acupuncture points such as LI4 or LI11 in the arms and ST36 or LR3 in the legs.

The standard dose of acupuncture needed for descending analgesia is shown in Table 9.2 – this can be applied in addition to any needles used for segmental analgesia, though still having respect for each individual person's sensitivity to acupuncture. Electrical stimulation is probably more effective than manual for activating this particular effect of acupuncture.

For a sustained effect in treating chronic pain, repeat the stimulus once or twice a week so that the benefit accumulates.

In deciding whether to use painful stimulation, we suggest readers should gain considerable experience before considering using it and select the patient carefully. The treatment has been described using ST37 for shoulder pain and LR3 for acute headache. The needle has to be stimulated strongly by hand, enough to be really uncomfortable. Of course patients need to be warned first and given the opportunity to abort the treatment if it becomes too strong for them.

Acupuncture analgesia for surgery

The combined effects of segmental and extrasegmental acupuncture stimulation have been used as the basis for acupuncture analgesia (hypoalgesia) for surgery. The increase in pain threshold that can be achieved by acupuncture in any particular patient varies greatly with many factors, including, for example, the particular circumstances and the susceptibility of the individual. While dramatic early reports from China showed major surgery apparently being conducted using acupuncture as the main form of analgesia, subsequent experience suggests that few individuals achieve sufficient increase in pain threshold to permit surgery, so it is used there with deep sedation and local analgesia. In Western practice, acupuncture analgesia when used alone for surgery is considered unreliable and not considered worthwhile as a sole intervention, though it has a clear role alongside conventional anaesthesia in postoperative pain relief.

Summary

The body's inbuilt system of analgesia, in which a centre in the midbrain (the periaqueductal grey, or PAG) suppresses nociception at the dorsal horn, can be stimulated by acupuncture. This descending inhibition may be effective just around the area where the stimulus is given or can under certain circumstances be activated more generally. The endogenous opioid β-endorphin has long been known to be at the heart of this analgesia, and at the dorsal horn level, serotonin and noradrenaline are key transmitters.

Further reading

Streitberger, K., Usichenko, T., 2016. Acupuncture analgesia for interventions. In: Filshie, J., White, A., Cummings, M. (Eds.), Medical Acupuncture: A Western Scientific Approach, second ed. Elsevier, Edinburgh, pp. 345–367.

A detailed, evidence-based discussion of history, mechanisms and applications of acupuncture analgesia in the operating room and similar locations.

CHAPTER 10

General effects II: central regulation

CONTENTS

Introduction

This chapter describes the effects of acupuncture on the non-cognitive aspects of brain function, including relaxation, mood and emotions, the autonomic system, various hormonal systems, and other central actions (e.g. nausea). We sum them up with the term *'central regulation'*, simply meaning that acupuncture's general effect is to restore homoeostasis. These effects are under the control of the parts of the brain other than the primary cortices (motor, sensory, visual, and auditory cortices); rather, they involve the *associative* cortex in various sites (such as prefrontal cortex and temporal cortex), deep brain structures (such as the limbic system and hypothalamus), and some parts of the brainstem (midbrain, pons and medulla).

One of the things that makes acupuncture satisfying for both patient and practitioner is any unexpected benefit from treatment. As well as the anticipated relief of pain – sometimes for the first time – patients also frequently report that they felt calm and relaxed, or even tired, and slept unusually well after treatment. This general improvement in well-being may be particularly valuable in starting the healing process in patients with chronic pain.

Occasionally, quite strong emotional reactions occur after acupuncture treatment, such as weeping, giggling and even anger. When you also take into account other rare events such as fainting, and very occasional reactions such as seizure or temporary comatose states, there is little doubt that acupuncture can influence some deep central brain functions.

A significant aspect of this benefit can be an improvement in *affect* or mood and in particular the emotional response to chronic pain. Chronic pain is not simply acute pain that is prolonged. It can be profoundly disturbing. A headache, for example, may incapacitate the patient more than the level of pain itself would seem to warrant. The role of the limbic system and deeper networks on affect, and their response to acupuncture, are becoming clearer.

The autonomic system is closely related to emotional and psychological responses. For example, essential hypertension is sometimes due to chronically raised sympathetic tone, and evidence is emerging that acupuncture can restore the tone towards normal. The ancient world view thought of life as a balance of opposing forces, so it is perhaps not surprising that acupuncture was said to 'restore the balance'.

The changes described in this chapter also explain how acupuncture may sometimes still be of some help to people whose symptoms cannot be treated but who gain psychologically from treatment. Of course, caution is needed because the effect may be due to the therapeutic relationship alone, bringing the risks of dependence; or it may be only short-lived, which can raise false hopes.

This interaction between psychology, emotion and acupuncture requires more analysis. Acupuncture is sometimes dismissed as 'just a placebo'. While acupuncture and the placebo response share some circuits and both involve release of endogenous transmitters such as opioid peptides, there is good evidence, as we see later, that there are different circuits and that acupuncture's central effects are greater than a placebo (Dhond et al., 2008). These are circuits where acupuncture interacts with the psychology of individual patients: it seems that a positive attitude to acupuncture is optimal – but not alone sufficient – for a response (Napadow et al., 2016). An empathic consultation helps, as may a fresh diagnosis, and perhaps simply the opportunity to lie still for 20 minutes with no responsibilities. But the needles themselves clearly contribute. We see the effects in training courses where students practise needling each other (in the context of training rather than therapy); some experience profound relaxation or tiredness after the training.

This effect seems not to need the use of specific point locations, though it may be more marked after needling well-known points (such as LI4, LR3). This again is noticed in acupuncture training courses, where drowsiness appears to be more common after needling the well-known classical points than after needling trigger points in muscle.

Readers will recall (Chapter 3) acupuncture's input into supraspinal structures from the anterolateral tract. We are concerned here with the group of fibres in this tract that project to the reticular formation in the brainstem, from where tertiary fibres project to the deep brain centres such as the limbic system. They provoke various central responses that are the subjects of this chapter.

Default mode network

Neurologists have known for many years that anatomical centres in the brain are linked to functions, such as memory, emotion, mood, etc. Recent advances in imaging, particularly functional MRI (fMRI), have revealed a higher level of functioning of the brain, the *functional networks*.

Each brain area has its own pattern of spontaneous, slow fluctuations, which can be identified with fMRI. The fluctuations change as the brain's function changes. Advanced methods of analysis have shown that these fluctuations may be synchronized between different centres. These centres can be regarded as functionally connected, forming *functional networks*.

Functional networks are linked to a particular activity, for example, auditory, visual, executive control or sensorimotor. But perhaps the most important network is active when the brain is not

---

Case History

A 41-year-old woman presented with severe, intermittent pain in the right axilla and forearm following lymph node dissection for breast cancer. She had marked lymphoedema on the right and was tender in the distribution of the intercostobrachial nerve.

She was treated with paraspinal points in the relevant segments (C7 to T4), tender points in infraspinatus, and LI4 on the L side only (to avoid needling the lymphoedematous arm). Six days after treatment she noticed galactorrhoea from the normal L breast. During the second treatment session, milk was again produced by the left breast. In view of this adverse event, treatment was abandoned. (Jenner, C., Filshie, J., 2002. AiM 20 (2–3), 107–8).

occupied with external tasks, hence it is called the 'default mode network (DMN)' (Buckner et al., 2008). It is a hallmark of daydreaming, rumination or self-reference. It is also active in people asked to recall memories or to think about other people's perspectives. The key components of the DMN are the *cingulate gyrus*, the *prefrontal cortex* and the *angular gyrus*, which is part of the *parietal lobe*.

In patients with chronic pain, the activity of the DMN becomes dysfunctional (Fig. 10.1). It is also disturbed in other conditions such as Alzheimer's and autism. Interestingly, acupuncture has been shown to improve the function of the DMN, compared with a placebo (Dhond et al., 2008). And trials have shown that a course of acupuncture can restore DMN connectivity to normal in patients with chronic pain due to fibromyalgia (Napadow et al., 2012) or low back pain (Li et al., 2014). The degree of improvement in DMN matched the degree of pain relief in individual patients.

There is some evidence that the network between DMN and the insula is particularly activated by acupuncture. This is relevant to pain control, since the insula projects onto the PAG and helps to activate descending inhibition (DI). Other areas closely linked to the DMN are components of the limbic system (see the following section) concerned with emotion, affect and certain cognitive functions such as decision-making.

The discovery of DMN and evidence supporting its role in chronic pain and its modification by acupuncture might provide a single, unifying explanation of acupuncture's central mechanisms in pain (Long et al., 2016).

The limbic system

Chapter 3 described how the *sensory/discriminatory* component of pain – its location, nature, quality and duration – is handled by the thalamus and the somatosensory cortex. The *emotional/affective* components involve the brainstem and subcortical networks, together with so-called 'associative' cortical areas such as the prefrontal and cingulate cortices, which make up the *limbic system*.

The definition of the limbic system is somewhat disputed. We use it here to include any brain centres that deal with the emotional/affective component of pain. The structures most involved in acupuncture are probably the amygdala, for memory and emotion; the hippocampus (and

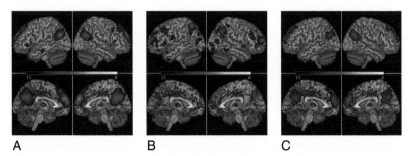

A   B   C

Figure 10.1 (A) The default mode networks (DMNs) of the healthy volunteers during rest comprised the inferior parietal lobule, posterior cingulate cortex and medial areas of the inferior, middle and superior frontal gyri, and the precuneus. (B) The DMN connectivities in patients with chronic low back pain (cLBP) before treatment were reduced in the dorsolateral prefrontal cortex, medial prefrontal cortex, anterior cingulate gyrus, and precuneus compared with the control group. (C) After treatment the DMNs of the patients with cLBP were almost identical to those of the control group. *(Reproduced with permission from Li, J., et al., 2014. Acupuncture treatment of chronic low back pain reverses an abnormal brain default mode network in correlation with pain relief. Acupuncture in Medicine, 32 (2), 102–108.)*

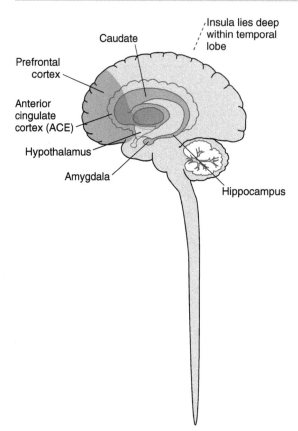

Figure 10.2 Limbic system: a schematic diagram of the main components.

TABLE 10.1 ■ Common effects of acupuncture on central structures (Chae et al., 2013)

Activation	Deactivation
Insula, thalamus, anterior cingulate cortex, somatosensory cortex, primary visual cortex, inferior frontal cortex, superior temporal cortex, superior temporal gyrus, and cerebellum[a]	Medial prefrontal cortex (mPFC), subgenual ACC, caudate, amygdala, posterior cingulate cortex (PCC), thalamus, parahippocampus, and cerebellum[a]

[a]Cerebellum is both activated and deactivated.

parahippocampus (para' = alongside)), for short-term memory; and the anterior cingulate cortex (ACC), for decision-making and for modulating the autonomic nervous system (see Fig. 10.2). The prefrontal cortex, insula and caudate are sometimes included. More structures are shown in Table 10.1.

The term 'limbic system' is used in this book to mean the parts of the brain that deal primarily with the emotional or affective aspects of pain.

Some authors use the term 'limbic-paralimbic-neocortical network (LPNN)' as an expansion of the limbic system to include the DMN. But until this is more widely accepted, we prefer *limbic system*.

The limbic system is closely linked with other structures relevant to the subconscious activity of the brain: the *nucleus accumbens*, which is regarded as the 'reward centre', is involved in pleasurable responses and therefore dependency behaviour such as drug abuse, and the hypothalamus, which is directly responsible for hormonal control and indirectly involved in modulating the autonomic nervous system.

Acupuncture activates some brain centres and deactivates others reasonably consistently, as shown in Table 10.1 (Chae et al., 2013). In general, the sensory pathway including insula and sensory cortex are activated, whereas the limbic system is deactivated. Evidence suggests that stronger deactivation is associated with greater relaxation.

Autonomic effects

Autonomic reflexes are of two types, *spinal* or *supraspinal*. Chapter 8 described the spinal autonomic reflexes in relation to bowel and bladder function. Now we discuss those functions that rely on the supraspinal autonomic reflexes. Acupuncture may have a role in reducing a chronically elevated central sympathetic output, which is a feature of some cases of hypertension, bladder dysfunction and polycystic ovary syndrome (PCOS).

While early studies did not show any long-term benefit of acupuncture for treating hypertension in unselected patients, it now seems clear that it can have an effect in patients where autonomic outflow is functionally disturbed (Cheng et al., 2015).

The same thing goes for other autonomic disturbances, such as functional bladder disorders. The decreased sympathetic tone can be reinforced by repeat treatment (Dyrehag et al., 1997). The role of acupuncture in other conditions that are sympathetic-dependent, such complex regional pain syndrome and Raynaud's disease, is still unclear, possibly because studies have not always used an appropriate type of stimulation.

Polycystic ovary syndrome (PCOS) is a condition much studied and includes infertility and metabolic syndrome. In some women with PCOS, sympathetic output is chronically elevated. Laboratory studies show that low-Hz EA can reduce sympathetic tone, as indeed can exercise. In related studies, low-Hz EA has also been shown to increase ovarian blood flow, which improved ovarian function in an animal model of PCOS (Stener-Victorin et al., 2009). These changes rely on supraspinal, not spinal, pathways. The effect is probably segmental, so the acupuncture should be given at the relevant segmental points.

MECHANISMS OF AUTONOMIC EFFECTS

The autonomic nuclei in the brainstem are under the control of the hypothalamus, which in turn is under regulation by the limbic system.

Low-frequency EA causes the release of neuropeptides centrally, together with serotonin, oxytocin and β-endorphin. The key control of autonomic output appears to be β-endorphin released from the hypothalamus (arcuate nucleus) and from the brainstem (nucleus tractus solitarius). The arcuate nucleus projects widely, including onto the autonomic centres, such as the cardiovascular centre (Stener-Victorin, 2016). The effect of β-endorphin is to inhibit the release of glutamate (GLU) in the autonomic centre, which is involved in increases in sympathetic outflow and raised blood pressure. Many other neurotransmitters are involved in the mechanisms.

The afferent pathways stimulate the arcuate nucleus of the hypothalamus to project downward to the autonomic centre in the medulla, and the descending tracts to segments controlling cardiac sympathetic output (T1-5, see Table 4.2 or 19.2).

CLINICAL APPLICATION FOR AUTONOMIC EFFECTS

Longhurst's group has explored point-specificity of these effects. Treatment to points in deep somatic structures such as median and peroneal nerves (PC5, PC6, ST36, ST37, LI4, LI10) modulates sympathetic output and reduces an elevated BP much more than points over superficial (cutaneous nerve) pathways (such as LI6, LI7, KI1, BL67) (Li et al., 2015).

For the kind of central autonomic effects we are discussing here, the research group showed that points should be treated bilaterally, but that using two pairs of points had no greater effect than one pair. Stimulation must be continued for at least 10 minutes to elicit the central response (brief stimulation may cause increased sympathetic output). Low-frequency EA shows much greater reduction of sympathetic output than high-frequency.

Stener-Victorin's group has also shown the value of low-frequency EA in modulating the supraspinal autonomic reflex (Stener-Victorin et al., 2004).

Hypothalamo–pituitary–adrenal axis

Acupuncture stimulation may influence the anterior pituitary gland via the hypothalamus. There is evidence that it stimulates the release into the circulation of both ACTH and β-endorphin, which are derived from a single precursor, proopiomelanocortin. How relevant the increased circulation of ACTH and β-endorphin after acupuncture are in clinical practice is not clear, since β-endorphin does not cross the blood-brain barrier. β-endorphin concentrations in the blood also respond to many non-specific stimuli, such as eating and exercise. It is important to distinguish between this β-endorphin circulating in the bloodstream and that which is released within the CNS around the periaqueductal grey.

Hypothalamo–pituitary–ovarian axis

The arcuate nucleus of the hypothalamus is the site for the so-called 'gonadotrophin (GnRH) pulse generator', so it is not unreasonable to predict that acupuncture may have some effect on release of GnRH. The clinical effects of this could include alteration in the regulation of menstrual timing and flow, and reduction of dysmenorrhoea. These effects on gonadotrophin-releasing hormone are now established, but the clinical effects, though reported widely as anecdotes, are not firmly supported by clinical trials.

Other endocrine effects

Postmenopausal hot flushes are due to dysfunction of the temperature regulatory centre, though the mechanisms are not fully understood. Some evidence suggests that release of β-endorphin in the hypothalamus tends to reduce the frequency of hot flushes, possibly by modifying the activity of CGRP, which is a potent vasodilator (Wyon et al., 1995), or by release of 5-HT, which has an effect on thermoregulation. Small clinical trials have suggested that acupuncture may reduce the incidence or severity of postmenopausal flushes, but it is still unclear whether this is more than an effect of expectation.

There are anecdotal reports that some patients find they need to alter their dose of insulin for a few days after having acupuncture. Acupuncture can affect glucose transport and insulin sensitivity, though there is little evidence that acupuncture can have any useful clinical effect on insulin-dependent diabetic patients.

The immune system

Acupuncture has been found in some studies to enhance the immune system. A potential immunomodulatory effect of acupuncture has long been mooted, but no plausible mechanism existed until Tracey reviewed the anti-inflammatory reflex (Tracey, 2002). Peripheral acetylcholine release, mediated principally by the vagus, can inhibit production of TNFα by splenic macrophages via the α7 nicotinic acetylcholine receptor (α7nAChR). Subsequently, it was discovered that the α7nAChR activated splenic noradrenergic fibres to reduce cytokine production from splenic macrophages (Vida et al., 2011). Tracey identified acupuncture as a potential method for increasing vagal tone along with direct vagal nerve stimulation.

A team in the United States published an experimental trial in a mouse model of sepsis that demonstrated a novel anti-inflammatory mechanism of indirect vagal stimulation (Torres-Rosas et al., 2014). The intervention they used was 10 minutes of EA to ST36, and it saved the majority of mice in the experiment from an otherwise fatal outcome. The effect of EA on TNF lasted for 72 hours after just 10 minutes of stimulation at ST36.

Since vagal stimulators are now starting to be used in patients with severe inflammatory arthropathies (Andersson and Tracey, 2012), it is tempting to wonder if self-applied EA to ST36 twice a week could have the same effect and ideally result in a reduction in frequency of inflammatory episodes.

The most comprehensive relevant clinical research in conditions in humans involves the rather common, and altogether less serious, condition allergic rhinitis. Acupuncture has been shown to produce significant benefit for patients with allergic rhinitis (mixed perennial and seasonal) (Brinkhaus et al., 2008, 2013)

Possible mechanisms include generalized or localized autonomic changes regulating the lymphoreticular system in the bone marrow and spleen, or circulation of β-endorphin, which induces immune changes through receptors on leucocytes. It is still not clear whether these effects of acupuncture are clinically relevant.

Drug dependency

Acupuncture has gained a reputation for helping addicts withdraw from their drugs. Acupuncture can reduce the excess dopamine production in the *nucleus accumbens,* which is the common pathway for addiction (Yoon et al., 2004) (see Fig. 10.3).

There are probably two separate clinical effects: a short-term reduction of the withdrawal symptoms (Han et al., 2011) and an improvement in the person's attitude and motivation, making them more likely to participate in the appropriate counselling and support services (Stuyt, 2014). Studies that simply test the effect on withdrawal alone have been disappointing, though they have often involved inadequate stimulation or used active control interventions (White, 2013).

Nausea and vomiting

Nausea and vomiting are centrally regulated, and acupuncture has been used in pregnancy, chemotherapy and postoperatively. These early studies have been followed by many others from different centres, generally confirming the effect (Lee et al., 2015). The sensation of nausea is a response of the emetic centre and chemoreceptor zones to a variety of stimuli.

Acupuncture, usually given at a point in the wrist (PC6), on the upper abdomen (CV12), or one below the knee (ST36), reduces the emetic response, but the precise mechanisms of action are still unknown.

General clinical application

The *nature* of the stimulus (the dose of acupuncture) may well be more relevant than *where* it is given. For general treatments in all conditions discussed in this chapter, it is best to treat bilaterally, using well-known points below the elbows and knees. Though body points are generally used for inducing central regulatory effects, auricular acupuncture may also be useful, as discussed in Chapter 17.

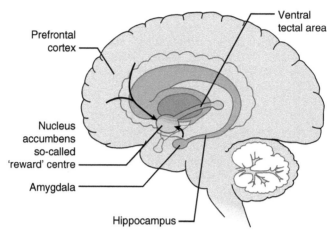

Figure 10.3   Relationships of the 'reward' centre or mesolimbic circuit of drug reinforcement. *(Reproduced with permission from, 2016., in: Ch 26. White A. Acupuncture for drug dependence and obesity. pp. 455–474. Filshie, J., White, A., Cummings, M. (Eds.), Medical Acupuncture: A Western Scientific Approach, Elsevier, Edinburgh second ed.)*

TABLE 10.2 ▉ **Points suitable for regulatory effects**

Arm Points	Leg Points
LI11 PC6 LI4	ST36 GB34 SP6 LR3

There is evidence that the effect of one needle on DMN can be increased by using more needles (Lin et al., 2016b). The points suggested in Table 10.2 can be needled down to muscle. It is convenient to treat points bilaterally.

To obtain these effects, avoid painful stimulation. Gentle manual stimulation to elicit *de qi* but avoiding pain is effective at inducing extensive limbic system deactivation (Fang et al., 2009; Lin et al., 2016b). Manual acupuncture, with manipulation, seems to alter the function of the DMN, and it is not yet clear whether EA is more or less effective (Huang et al., 2012). It may be sensible to consider EA if there is no response to manual stimulation. After inserting the needles, let the patient relax quietly for 10–30 minutes without disturbance.

To maximize these central effects, it seems important to ensure that the nervous system is appropriately 'primed' before treatment. This means that the patient should be relaxed, confident, warm and comfortable, and pain should be avoided when needling.

It is difficult to predict the response of any individual patient, so practitioners must learn to observe carefully how the patient responds and to adjust the dose of acupuncture accordingly. Responses can be powerful, and practitioners should be aware of unwanted emotional effects. Patients who appear in any way emotionally unstable should be treated particularly carefully, and a course of treatment should not be prolonged in these patients if their condition does not respond quickly.

SHAM ACUPUNCTURE AND THE AFFECTIVE COMPONENT OF PAIN

Interestingly, there is rather good evidence that a convincing form of sham acupuncture (using blunt needles, but suggesting to the patient that this is an active treatment) can produce distinct changes in the limbic system. It seems highly probable that the type III fibres usually stimulated by acupuncture are not involved in conveying this effect, and it is much more likely that this effect of sham acupuncture on the limbic system is a result of touch activating the C tactile fibre system (Lund and Lundeberg, 2006). These aspects of treatment could be described as the pleasantness of acupuncture. With genuine acupuncture, when needles are inserted and stimulated in an appropriate way, there is an additional effect that seems to involve the insula very specifically (Pariente et al., 2005).

One interpretation of the evidence from imaging studies is that the affective component of pain will respond to any form of acupuncture that stimulates the limbic system, whereas the sensory component of pain is likely to respond better to segmental analgesia. The limbic system can be stimulated by rather non-specific needling, whereas segmental analgesia depends more on stimulating in the appropriate segment.

This non-specific effect creates quite a problem for 'placebo' controls in clinical trials. This difference could explain the findings of the large series of clinical trials in Germany in the early 2000s: acupuncture and sham acupuncture have similar effects on migraine, tension headache and back pain, whereas for knee pain segmental acupuncture is significantly superior to sham acupuncture. The explanation that has been proposed is that migraine, tension headache and back pain have a high affective component, which responds to non-specific needle stimulation (Lund and Lundeberg, 2006). In contrast, knee pain is mainly sensory, so specific analgesic effects are required.

The affective component of pain is rarely measured in clinical trials, but at least one study has found that patients who have received acupuncture report that the affective component is reduced more than the sensory component (Thomas et al., 1991). Patients may still have their chronic pain, but it bothers them less.

Summary

Acupuncture may have effects on non-cognitive aspects of brain function, including relaxation, mood and emotions, as well as on autonomic and hormonal systems. This may add a useful dimension to treatment of chronic pain. Brain imaging studies have shown responses in particular locations, including the limbic system, and on particular functions, including the default mode network. These effects extend to recorded effects on the immune system, for example, in allergic rhinitis and on nausea and vomiting.

Further reading

Stener-Victorin, E., 2016. Acupuncture and the autonomic nervous system. In: Filshie, J., White, A., Cummings, M. (Eds.), Medical Acupuncture: A Western Scientific Approach, second ed. Elsevier, Edinburgh.
   A thorough description of the mechanism and role of acupuncture in modulating visceral, endocrine and metabolic function.

CHAPTER 11

Traditional Chinese acupuncture reinterpreted

Introduction

The previous chapters have described approaches to acupuncture that are consistent with current knowledge of anatomy, physiology and pathology. Why do we now describe the traditional views? Partly because we want to add to the discussion on how acupuncture in traditional Chinese medicine (TCM) may have developed in the first place, partly because we believe patients should be aware of the basis of the acupuncture treatment given by a traditional Chinese acupuncture (TCA) practitioner, and partly because we think there may be aspects of TCA that still have something to offer.

'Acupuncture' (literally, 'acus' = needle + 'pungere' to puncture or prick, from the Latin) is a European word that is an attempt to represent the Chinese *zhen-jiu*, which means 'needle and moxa' therapy (Birch and Kaptchuk, 1999; Lu and Needham, 1980; Schnorrenberger, 2003). TCA deserves the respect due to any therapy that has such a long history of a consistent, structured, and academic approach. Acupuncture and traditional Chinese herbal medicine remain the treatment of choice for some populations, at least for some conditions.

But there is a difference between respect and unquestioning acceptance. TCM is still taught and practised using models and methods that have not been updated in the light of scientific discoveries, in the way that Hippocratic medicine has. We think that is a problem and a weakness. As we shall see, the approach to acupuncture was continually updated for centuries in the light of new information about the structure and function of the body. Why should that process stop now? We believe Western medical acupuncture is simply the latest chapter in an evolving story.

While the Chinese theories of acupuncture may be attractive and 'real' in the sense of apparently explaining symptoms, they often appear outdated and even incorrect to someone trained in health care in the scientific era. Learning TCA involves suspending one's natural critical appraisal, which someone who is trained in health care is unlikely to want to do. This chapter, which is unavoidably superficial, attempts to describe some of the concepts of TCM and to point out some of its deficiencies; it is very much a personal view.

Chinese origins of acupuncture

The idea that acupuncture originated in China about 2000 years ago is widely accepted. However, it may be only partially correct, as we discuss throughout this chapter.

The first known text on acupuncture is the *Huang Di Nei Jing,* or *The Yellow Emperor's Classic of Internal Medicine* (Veith, 1949), which is said to date from 200–100 BC. This detailed work describes systems of diagnosis and treatment with herbs and needles, though does not name acupuncture points. The text of the *Yellow Emperor's Internal Classic* is likely to be a compilation of traditions that had evolved over preceding years (Kaplan, 1997). The information is presented in the form of questions posed by the emperor and answered by his minister, Chhi-Po. Medical problems are discussed in terms of the Taoist world view, which was prevalent at the time. This text is regarded as the founding canon of Chinese medicine, rather in the way that Hippocrates' works were the foundation of Western medicine (Kaptchuk, 1983). However, unlike Hippocrates' work, the text is still used as treatment guidelines.

Modern readers find it difficult to embrace the full meaning of the text because of the remoteness of culture and concepts. Often an intuitive explanation turns out to be quite wrong; for example, the meridians could be thought of as lines connecting acupuncture points. However the meridians came first, as documents found in a burial tomb dating from 168 BC refer to a system of meridians but not points (Chen, 1997).

European origins of acupuncture

Prehistoric human remains have produced tantalizing evidence that acupuncture may have originated in Europe. Ötzi the 'Tyrolean Ice Man' was a hunter whose body was preserved in an Alpine glacier in about 3300 BC, emerging from the melting face in 1991 (Dorfer et al., 1998). Ötzi's body carries 47 tattoo marks, organized in 15 groups, mainly on the back and legs (Plates 6A and B). The tattoos consist of spots or lines of charcoal deposited in the subcutaneous layer of the skin. Because they are situated in areas that would be covered in clothes, and because of their shape, these tattoos do not seem to have the same purpose as most tattoos from that era – decoration or ritual. Instead, it has been suggested that they have some medical purpose and may be signs of cautery, which is a common feature of folk medicine (Nogier, 1981).

Dorfer was interested in Ötzi's tattoos and was inspired to consult some acupuncture experts about them (Dorfer et al., 1999). After careful measurements, these experts concluded that 9 of the 15 groups of tattoos lie within a few millimetres of classical acupuncture points. Even more suggestively, their locations are the same as the points that traditional Chinese acupuncturists might have used to treat the medical conditions that x-ray film and other examinations showed Ötzi to have had at the time he died: bladder meridian points on the back and the leg for spinal degeneration; and LR8, SP6 and GB points for an intestinal problem – infestation with worms.

Ötzi's tattoos, therefore, suggest that a system of treatment that was remarkably similar to Chinese acupuncture existed in Europe long before any evidence of it in China. While this interpretation is speculative, it challenges the idea that the Chinese had a monopoly on acupuncture.

The evolution of acupuncture in China

Acupuncture continued to evolve over the centuries that followed its description in the *Yellow Emperor's Internal Classic,* and in some areas it was regarded as routine therapy together with herbs, massage, diet and moxibustion (heat). About the end of the first millennium, Wang Wei-Yi (987–1067) constructed hollow bronze statues (Plate 7) that clearly depicted acupuncture points as holes (Ma, 1992). During the Ming Dynasty (1368–1644), *The Great Compendium of Acupuncture and Moxibustion* was published, giving clear descriptions of 361 points that form the basis of modern acupuncture.

Acupuncture was not practised everywhere in China, and the approach to treatment was far from uniform throughout the country (Birch and Kaptchuk, 1999). Many different esoteric theories of diagnosis and treatment emerged, sometimes even contradicting each other, largely due to vast distances between centres and lack of communication that resulted in local traditions. Rival acupuncture schools tried to establish their exclusiveness and influence.

Interest in acupuncture declined from the 17th century onwards as it came to be regarded as superstitious and irrational in comparison to Western medicine (Baldry, 1993; Ma, 1992). Acupuncture was finally excluded from the Imperial Medical Institute by decree of the emperor in 1822. The knowledge and skill were retained, however, both as an interest among academics and as a therapy among rural healers. The final ignominy for acupuncture arrived in 1929 when it was outlawed, along with other forms of TCM (Ma, 1992).

After the installation of the Communist government in 1949, traditional forms of medicine, including acupuncture, were reinstated, possibly out of both national pride and sheer practicality: low-cost medicine was the only means of providing even basic levels of health care to the massive population. Mao Tse-tung promoted TCM with the words, 'Let a thousand flowers flourish'– though it is reported that Mao himself rejected acupuncture for his illnesses and used Western medicine (Basser, 1999).

During this renaissance of traditional healing, an attempt was made to form a consensus of all the divergent strands of herbal medicine, acupuncture and moxibustion, and to produce a unified version of TCM (Birch and Kaptchuk, 1999). TCM became available in Western-style hospitals in China, though not in the same departments as Western medicine. At about the same time, acupuncture research institutes were established and several researchers in China sought more rational explanations of acupuncture, such as Ji-Sheng Han in Beijing, who undertook ground-breaking research on the release of neurotransmitters (Han and Terenius, 1982).

The worldwide spread of acupuncture

Through China's influence on its neighbours, Korea and Japan assimilated acupuncture and herbal medicine around the 6th century (Baldry, 1993) and both countries still use these therapies, often in parallel with Western medicine. Acupuncture arrived in Vietnam when commercial routes opened up in the 8th–10th centuries. In the West, France was one of the first countries to adopt acupuncture (Kaplan, 1997). Reports of acupuncture were brought back by Jesuit missionaries from the 16th century onwards. Willem Ten Rhijne was the first Western doctor to write a description of acupuncture in about 1680. He was a physician to the East India Company and witnessed acupuncture practice in Japan (Bivens, 2000). The practice was embraced by some French clinicians. Berlioz, father of the composer, ran clinical trials on acupuncture and wrote papers on it in 1816 (Bivens, 2000). The French style of acupuncture was deeply influenced by a diplomat, Soulier de Morant, who spent many years in China and published a number of treatises on the subject of acupuncture from 1939 onwards.

In the first half of the 19th century, there was a flurry of interest in America and Britain, and a number of publications appeared in the scientific literature, including an editorial article in the *Lancet* entitled 'Acupuncturation' (Anon., 1823). But by the middle of the 19th century, acupuncture was no longer of interest, though it was briefly resurrected in one edition of Sir William Osler's textbook of medicine (Osler, 1912). He suggested that acupuncture was the best treatment for acute lumbago, and any needle would do, even a lady's hatpin!

THE 20TH CENTURY

In 1971, James Reston, a senior reporter for the *New York Times*, was visiting China in preparation for President Nixon's visit. He required emergency surgery for appendicitis, and during the recovery period he developed paralytic ileus, which was treated with acupuncture. He described the experience in his influential column (Reston, 1971) and subsequently several teams of US physicians made fact-finding tours of China to assess acupuncture. They were particularly interested in its use for surgical analgesia, though they eventually concluded that acupuncture was not reliable as a sole analgesic. Their reports stimulated a number of research studies, particularly in treating experimental pain in volunteers. Acupuncture finally gained a certain amount of respectability in the United States after the positive conclusions of a National Institutes of Health (NIH) consensus conference (NIH Consensus Development Panel, 1998).

Individual doctors from the UK also visited China to see acupuncture for themselves and made a persistent effort to reconsider the traditional explanations of acupuncture in scientific terms (Baldry, 2005a), as discussed in the Introduction.

We shall now briefly describe a selection of the traditional concepts and speculate on how they might have arisen.

Traditional Chinese acupuncture theories

THE CONTEXT OF TRADITIONAL CHINESE ACUPUNCTURE

Acupuncture was practised in China as part of medicine, together with herbs, massage and dietary manipulation. Presumably, Chinese doctors had to deal with the typical major diseases common to any early civilization, including major infections, such as tuberculosis, acute sepsis, meningitis and abscesses; congenital disorders and deformities; chronic conditions such as heart failure or hyper- and hypothyroidism; trauma and fractures; as well as acute surgical emergencies. Strong and invasive treatments were developed, and it is interesting to compare early medicine in the West, which used drastic treatments such as bloodletting and purgation. The development of the germ theory and subsequent provision of clean water and sanitation changed the face of medicine.

There is no single theory of traditional acupuncture, and even the attempt in the 1950s to unify it into TCM fails to satisfy all practitioners. It seems that some physicians would just treat symptoms and signs, but others also wanted to know about the constitution of the individual as a prerequisite (Kaptchuk, 1983). They would take into account the patient's preferences for one kind of weather or another, the colour of their skin, their favourite foods, or the time of year of the onset of symptoms. Disease was seen as an integral and perhaps inevitable part of a person's very existence rather than a condition produced by a single identifiable cause.

Chinese approaches to acupuncture use various combinations of the following basic concepts.

CHINESE ANATOMY AND PHYSIOLOGY

It is important to credit the ancient Chinese physicians with some remarkable discoveries; their understanding of the structure and function of the body was an impressive achievement for its day, well in advance of Western anatomy and physiology at the time. They provided some great insights, such as the central importance of the liver for body metabolism and (probably) the concept of circulation of the blood. However, China was largely isolated from the scientific revolution in Europe, so the impact of the scientific understanding of anatomy and physiology on TCM was very limited (Kendall, 2002).

Briefly, the Chinese considered that human physiology consists of the interaction of three vital substances – qi, Blood and Body fluids. Qi is the most fundamental of these: humans were born with 'hereditary qi', which is stored in the kidneys and maintained by food and air so that it could circulate to nourish and defend the body. When qi becomes 'pathological'– deficiency, stagnation, rebellion, for example – then symptoms arise and disease follows. At the risk of oversimplifying, deficiency of *qi* means cold, underactivity or weakness; stagnation is probably equivalent to muscle spasm; and rebellion is exemplified by vomiting. Blood is a 'highly condensed' form of *qi* and inseparable from it. Body fluids derive from food: pure fluids enter the body and the impure fluids are secreted via the urinary tract. Blood and body fluids can have disturbances of their own, which must be diagnosed and corrected.

Throughout this description, one can perceive the efforts of intelligent minds working out a theoretical explanation for their careful observations of man in health and disease. It is tempting to speculate how the Chinese derived their particular explanations for the structure and function of the body, and we shall give just three examples:

1. In TCM, the internal organs are classified as either solid or hollow. Oddly, both Lung and Heart were regarded as solid. Could physicians have been misled by the solid appearance of these organs at *postmortem* examination?
2. In TCM the Heart is regarded as the 'seat of the mind' (Shenmen). Did this reflect the observation that the Heart races when we become excited or afraid? Was the Heart assumed to be the seat of both the racing pulse and the excitement?
3. In TCM the Spleen was involved in the absorption of food: food enters the stomach, and an explanation had to be found for how it combines with air, in the lungs. Was it assumed to pass along the most obvious route – through the Spleen and then through the diaphragm? Naturally the diaphragm had to be perforated – which is exactly how it was perceived in Western medicine before Harvey's time.

Traditional acupuncturists still think of the Spleen as being closely associated with the stomach and digestion, which is far from the truth as we know it. When challenged, they say they think of the Spleen as a 'function' rather than a physical organ: the function attributed to the Spleen is transportation of food and fluids. This idea, which seems odd to modern minds, becomes compounded when TCM says that a 'deficiency of the Spleen' causes peripheral oedema, and the deficiency arises from an invasion of 'Dampness' (Maciocia, 1989), for example, from sitting on damp surfaces.

QI

Qi (pronounced as 'chee' in cheese) is a term used in acupuncture with two rather different meanings:

- *Qi* includes the sense of activity, or the potential for action. It is the difference between life and death, between still and sparkling water. It is similar to what is understood in physics as kinetic, potential or metabolic energy. Humans are considered to be born with an allocation of *qi* and to replenish it with food and air, so that the *qi* can be distributed throughout the body as 'nourishment' and 'defence'. Disease arises when *qi* is disturbed; this can be an excess, a deficiency, or a blockage. This seems a reasonable approach to describing what we would know as (1) the supply of tissue nutrients such as oxygen and glucose, and (2) tissue repair and various immune functions.
- *Qi* is also sometimes used in the abstract sense of the Life Force in 'energetic medicine'. This is probably a misunderstanding, which we shall not discuss further here (Kendall, 2002; Schnorrenberger, 2003; Soulié de Morant, 1957).

YIN/YANG 'BALANCE'

Another fundamental concept in TCA is the balance of opposites, represented as *yin* and *yang*. The original meanings of these words are the dark and light sides of a hill: *yin* is dark, cold and inactive, whereas *yang* is bright, hot and active. Sick people are considered to have an imbalance of *yin* and *yang*, and treatment is designed to rebalance them.

This concept is similar to Claude Bernard's *milieu internal,* that is, what we understand as homoeostasis – though of course many centuries older. It is easy to find examples in medicine where physiology involves 'balance' and disease involves the loss of this balance, either as the cause or as the effect: temperature regulation; autonomic control of skin blood flow; gastrointestinal motility; thyrotoxicosis and hypothyroidism; hyper- and hypocorticosteroid conditions. But that does not mean that every medical condition can be seen as a disturbance of balance; infectious diseases, cancer, degenerative diseases and fractures, for example, cannot be explained in this way.

We speculate that one original – and very sound – observation came to be applied as a general rule in every situation: *yin/yang* balance evolved to become the vital basis of good health. The Chinese seemed to excel in making general rules out of accurate observations, and we shall see other examples of this tendency.

FIVE PHASES (ELEMENTS)

The concept of five 'phases' is very ancient. The word translated as 'phases' has no exact equivalent in English and is often translated as 'elements', though it is more elaborate than the four elements of Greek or medieval European medicine: Earth, Air, Fire and Water (Maciocia, 1989). It has nothing to do with the 'elements' of the periodic table. The concept behind the five phases is complex: everything – whether physical object, animal or human being – was thought to comprise five phases in every aspect of its existence: Wood, Fire, Earth, Metal and Water. Each of the phases has corresponding features in every aspect of life, for example, the type of emotional character, colour, season, direction and flavour. Thus Wood corresponds with anger, the colour green, spring, the East and sour flavour. Moreover, each phase is also linked to a pair of organs – Wood, for example, is linked with Liver and Gall Bladder. So an upset in any of the phases would cause disease in these particular organs and could be influenced by needling the meridians of the same name.

Each phase predominates at a different period of the day in a fixed cycle. Each phase influences the other phases, stimulating the one immediately following it and inhibiting the one following that (Fig. 11.1) (Lawson-Wood and Lawson-Wood, 1973).

Because the concept of five phases is circular, and everything relates to everything else, a practitioner can always argue that one single fault somewhere in the system has produced all the subsequent faults. All conditions are explicable as extensions of one fundamental imbalance. This gives an impression of holism but is unconvincing.

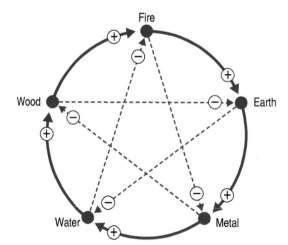

Figure 11.1 Diagram of the cycle of five phases, indicating interrelationships: each phase supposedly stimulates the next (e.g. Water, Wood) and inhibits the subsequent one (e.g. Water, Fire).

MERIDIANS

The Chinese used the word *jing-luo* to describe a bundle of vessels, channels or meridians. Some authorities argue that these were palpable physical structures; almost certainly what we now know as blood vessels, nerves and tendons (Schnorrenberger, 2003).

When the concept of fixed acupuncture points developed, there seems to have been a quite separate idea of meridians that were used as an *aide memoir* for finding them – rather as, in modern astronomy, the constellations are used to remember the position of the stars. Even if the stars themselves are unrelated, their position can be remembered from where they appear in relation to the other stars.

The concept of meridians was used in various ways in clinical practice:

- Diseases 'invaded' the meridian, that is, superficial symptoms would lead to damage of the associated organ – unless they were repulsed by acupuncture.
- Needling of the meridians would improve the condition of the associated organ.
- In the five-phases approach, each meridian was supposed to have 'control points' that directly influenced the meridians of the other phases.
- Points at the end of a meridian were needled to treat a painful condition elsewhere on the meridian.

ACUPUNCTURE POINTS

We discussed the concepts of acupuncture points, and possible explanations of their origin, in Chapter 4.

ASSOCIATED EFFECT POINTS

The Bladder meridians (one on each side of the body) run down alongside the spine and onwards down the back of the legs. As the meridians run about 4 cm from the midline, over the longitudinal muscles, classical points are shown at almost every spinal segmental level. Some of these have come to be associated with having an effect on one or other of the organs. Interestingly, the associated organ is innervated by that segmental level, as discussed under viscerotomes in Chapter 4 and shown in Figure 11.2. This suggests that the Chinese approach to acupuncture does actually acknowledge biomedical concepts.

Diagnosis in traditional Chinese medicine

TONGUE DIAGNOSIS

TCM practitioners may inspect the tongue carefully for its colouring and texture, looking at the margins of the tongue and the body. They use information from the tongue in forming a diagnosis. Now, some clinical conditions, such as severe iron-deficiency anaemia, acute streptococcal infection, or local Candida infection, do show distinctive and even florid changes in the appearance of the tongue. It seems possible that these known associations in a few particular cases have been extended to make a general rule – that the tongue always provides information in making a diagnosis.

PULSE DIAGNOSIS

TCA practitioners often study the pulse in great detail and claim to glean much more information from it than Western physicians do. Some say it gives information on the state of the meridians (e.g., Liver deficiency); others use a general description ('slippery' pulse). It is a common observation

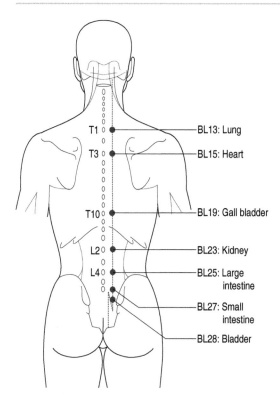

T1 — BL13: Lung
T3 — BL15: Heart
T10 — BL19: Gall bladder
L2 — BL23: Kidney
L4 — BL25: Large intestine
BL27: Small intestine
BL28: Bladder

Figure 11.2 The 'associated effect points' of traditional Chinese acupuncture, demonstrating a biomedical understanding of the segmental innervation of the viscera.

that some conditions do produce highly typical abnormalities in the strength, rhythm or nature of the pulse: the water-hammer pulse of aortic incompetence or the thready pulse of shock, for example. Again, the examination of the pulse seems to have been elevated into something central to making a diagnosis in every condition.

THE NATURE OF TRADITIONAL CHINESE MEDICINE DIAGNOSIS

TCM has a remarkable ability to allow apparently contradictory ideas to coexist. Some authors state that diseases are not 'caused' but are an essential and inevitable component of the individual's pattern (Kaptchuk, 1983), while others discuss the causes of disease, just like Western medicine does. Acupuncturists may use terms such as external pathogenical factors, or internal emotional influences such as excessive worry, or behaviour such as an unbalanced diet, or excess of sexual activity as the causes of an illness. Some practitioners will work with the concept of five phases, whereas others will use the modern TCM concept of 'syndromes' (i.e. relatively constant pattern of symptoms and a formula for treating them). For example, a stiff and painful neck with rapid onset and changeable symptoms might be due to pathogenical 'Wind' (Maciocia, 1989). This is summed up as the idea of 'root and branch' treatment. Root treatment is supposed to address the patient's fundamental 'imbalance', but branch treatment only deals with the symptoms.

Table 11.1 shows a list of some of the diagnostic approaches that can be used (), separately or together, to explain the symptoms that any particular patient presents.

These diagnostic methods of TCM need to be tested for reliability, in the sense that different practitioners applying them to particular patients should agree on the diagnosis. We would not be surprised if there is some agreement because, after all, they are systematic methods of classifying

TABLE 11.1 ■ **Examples of traditional diagnostic methods**

Diagnostic method	Explanation and/or example
Five phases	Imbalance of one (or more) elements (e.g. dizziness and headaches from insufficient Wood)
Organ syndrome	Symptoms due to disturbance of an organ's function, such as lassitude and loose stools from Spleen deficiency
Disturbance in *Qi*, Blood or Body fluids	What we might refer to as internal medicine (e.g. nausea and vomiting due to 'rebellious *Qi*'
Eight principles	Diagnosis by Interior/Exterior, Hot/Cold, Full/Empty, and *Yin/Yang* character of the disease (e.g. pale face, tiredness and lack of appetite from Empty *Qi*)
Meridians and collaterals	Symptoms explained by the pathway of a meridian (e.g. the symptoms of vaginal discharge, cold feeling along the meridian and leg pain indicate a disturbance of the Spleen meridian)
Pathogenical factors, from the climate	Aversion to cold, sneezing and runny nose due to an invasion of Wind

medical symptoms and signs. For example, the TCA diagnoses made in women with 'idiopathic' infertility (i.e. cause unknown to Western medicine) showed some reliability in distinguishing them from those with other causes (Coyle and Smith, 2005). It does not follow that TCA diagnosis is 'reliable' in the sense of confirming, for example, that Spleen deficiency is a meaningful diagnosis in a case of vaginal discharge.

We accept that TCM diagnosis may be able to make more subtle differentiations between types of patients than the diagnostic methods of Western medicine. For example, Western doctors may talk about different 'types' of patients but do not have a terminology or system for codifying them. This is an aspect of TCM that could be well worth exploring in some detail.

Traditional Chinese treatment

POINT SELECTION

In classical TCM the acupuncturist selects the points according to their actions, matching these points exactly to the individual patient's diagnosis. Here are three examples from a standard text (Maciocia, 1989):
- BL62 (just below the external malleolus) 'benefits the eyes, relaxes sinews, clears the mind and eliminates interior Wind'.
- SP10 (just above the knee) 'cools the Blood, regulates menstruation'.
- LI11 (lateral border of elbow) 'expels exterior Wind, clears Heat, resolves Dampness and benefits the sinews and joints'.

One can only speculate on how these particular activities ever became attached to individual points; presumably, it was a result of observing the general effects we have discussed in Chapter 5 and some creative interpretation.

The use of this rationale for choosing points for needling seems to us to be a central and significant problem in applying TCM. This is a fundamentally important principle of TCM that is desperately awaiting some kind of supporting evidence.

NEEDLE MANIPULATION

In line with the idea of influencing the flow of qi in the meridian, some practitioners use particular needle manipulations, such as clockwise or anticlockwise rotation and strong as opposed to gentle, supposedly to increase ('reinforce') or decrease ('drain') the *qi*. While the speed of rotation could stimulate nerve endings differentially, it is difficult to imagine that opposite directions of rotation have different effects. After removing the needle, some acupuncturists place their finger over the hole, 'to stop the *qi* escaping'.

CLAIMS OF HOLISM

Traditional acupuncturists generally claim that they are practising 'holistically', because their diagnosis can take account of a variety of factors in the patient, such as their food preferences, frequency of sexual intercourse, and the effect of weather on the symptoms. However, holistic medicine is truly a function of the overall approach of the practitioner, not of any system of medicine. There is nothing inherently more holistic in TCA diagnosis than in a comprehensive Western medical assessment. In fact, a good Western medical assessment may well be more holistic in taking greater account of psychological and social factors in a case, which hardly feature in TCA. No system of medicine can claim a monopoly on holism.

Traditional Chinese and Western medical acupuncture

The traditional theories of acupuncture have been challenged in the West by various authors in the United Kingdom (Baldry, 1993; Campbell, 2001; Filshie and White, 1998; Mann, 1992) and the United States (Ulett, 1992). We limit ourselves to some general observations and some rather speculative comments.

Despite a considerable amount of research to try to explain the *meridians* or channels – as nerves, electrical pathways, conduits of sound, pathways in the collagen matrix – there is no evidence to support their existence as physical structures. They are much better explained as a way of understanding common clinical observations, such as pain from nerve-root entrapment like sciatica, pressure on other nerves like the greater occipital nerve, referred sensations from trigger points, or the red lines of ascending lymphangitis, as well as propagated needle sensation that is likely to be due to spinal-cord interconnections. Symptom patterns in one region may have generated the idea that meridians run throughout the body to make a complete and coherent pattern.

There are many concepts in classical acupuncture which can easily be understood as a way of interpreting everyday observations in different terminology. For example, diseases are considered to first invade superficially and then, if unchecked, to invade the internal organs. This could simply reflect observations such as:

- a cold starts in the nose and throat; it may lead to pneumonia in the lungs
- with increasing age, musculoskeletal conditions become more common; serious internal diseases follow later – such as heart attacks, tuberculosis or cancer.

Similarly, back pain is commonly attributed to 'stagnation of *qi* in the Kidneys'. Stagnation of *qi* is probably what we would call muscle spasm, and in patients with back pain, spasm often occurs where the kidneys are situated. This diagnosis of stagnation may be little more than a description of what is observed and not an indication of kidney disease. These concepts serve to reinforce the convictions of classical TCM acupuncturists, but they cannot be used to provide an argument in favour of classical acupuncture when they can be explained perfectly rationally.

Some more general comments can be added here about the classical (Chinese) interpretation of acupuncture. One problem with acupuncture is that so many different forms of diagnosis are still used, long after the world view on which they are based has been discarded. Different schools of TCA seem to differ in their treatment approaches but probably all have very similar results in clinical practice. Given what we now know about the widespread effects of stimulating the body

TABLE 11.2 ■ **A summary of the principal differences between Western medical acupuncture and traditional Chinese acupuncture**

Traditional Chinese acupuncture	Western medical acupuncture
Theory	
Acts on *qi*	Acts on nerve and muscle
Corrects underlying imbalances	Cannot treat the underlying cause of diseases
'Meridians' are of fundamental importance, and their names are meaningful	Meridian names are only useful labels
High regard for accumulated clinical traditions	High regard for empirical evidence
Integrates new understandings into the old	Self-correcting, rejecting ideas when they become obsolete
Indication	
Effective for any condition	Effective only for certain types of condition
Practice	
Traditional Chinese diagnosis	Conventional Western diagnosis
Points precisely located	Points are general guidelines to appropriate stimulation sites
Individualized therapy, emphasis on point stimulation	Individualized therapy, emphasis mostly on location

with a needle anywhere within quite a large area, it seems that the only rational conclusion is that the actual traditional diagnosis is probably not that important, but that stimulating the patient with a needle is.

Seen from the Western, scientific perspective, acupuncture seems to be a relatively straightforward therapy, given our knowledge of the structure and function of the body. It seems unnecessary to complicate it with elaborate theories. The Western approach to acupuncture is often dismissed as an oversimplification of the original therapy, limited to the treatment of symptoms. Classical acupuncture in contrast claims to 'correct fundamental imbalances' (Table 11.2). We have seen no evidence to convince us that this 'correction of fundamental imbalances' is any more than a combination of generalized beneficial effects on brain centres (as discussed in Chapter 6) together with the patient's expectation of success. Many ancient descriptions of acupuncture actually seem to regard it as treatment of symptoms, not the root cause (Birch and Kaptchuk, 1999). Even the *Yellow Emperor's Classic of Internal Medicine* stated that acupuncture was really only suitable for superficial symptoms and that internal diseases required herbs. The way we apply acupuncture may actually be more in line with ancient tradition than the TCM approach!

Finally, there is the manner in which the understanding of a therapy grows over time. Traditional acupuncture evolved through the unchallenged opinions of experts. It was assumed that these experts had gained accurate knowledge and deep understanding from a lifetime of self-critical observation and experiment. This assumption is probably wrong, since according to our current understanding of 'clinical impressions' compared with 'evidence-based medicine', the so-called 'medical experts' are often wrong.

We prefer to understand as well as we can now, but to be prepared to ditch our ideas when new evidence comes along.

Summary

Acupuncture is recorded from China about 2000 years ago, but a similar practice may have existed in Europe approximately 5000 years ago. The Chinese traditional practice varied over geography and time, and evolved over many centuries during many changes of world views, retaining concepts from each period. In China, acupuncture was gradually rejected in favour of Western medicine from the 17th century, but interest was restored from the 1950s.

Traditional concepts include *qi, yin* and *yang*, five phases (elements), and meridians. Traditional Chinese understanding of structure and function was impressive in its day but has not changed in the light of scientific discoveries and appears outdated and erroneous. Diagnosis in traditional Chinese acupuncture may use several models at the same time, and treatment relies on activating the specific properties that points are supposed to have. A rational approach based on knowledge obtained scientifically can explain many of the concepts of TCM.

Further reading

Kendall, D.E., 2002. Dao of Chinese Medicine: Understanding an Ancient Healing Art. Oxford, New York.
This book claims to show the truth (Dao) about traditional Chinese medicine by reinterpreting the Chinese explanations in the light of subsequent biomedical discoveries. It is stimulating and knowledgeable, even though some find it ultimately unconvincing, and recommended reading for anyone interested in exploring the field.
Lu, G.D., Needham, J., 2002. Celestial Lancets: A History and Rationale of Acupuncture and Moxa. Routledge Curzon, London.
This work is part of a major project of enormous breadth and scholarship called 'Science and Civilisation' in China to which the authors devoted their lives at the Needham Institute in Cambridge. It is essential and very accessible reading for anyone seriously interested in Chinese medicine. The original publication in 1980 has been republished with an introduction by Vivienne Lo, which discusses research since 1980, including texts discovered since the 1970s, and suggests ways in which the original interpretations may need to be modified. For example, needling the body was originally associated with lancing abscesses; the idea that sharp stones were the forerunner of acupuncture with needles is shown to be far from convincing, and the theoretical foundation of acupuncture and moxibustion could not have occurred before the first century BC. However, as Lo herself comments, the original text is 'unlikely to be superseded'.
Schnorrenberger, C., 2003. Chen-Chiu, the Original Acupuncture: A New Healing Paradigm. Wisdom Publications, Somerville, Massachusetts.
The author is a German physician who has been studying Chinese medicine since the 1970s and has published a number of works in German and English. This book is a summary of his approach to Chinese medicine, in particular the way that he believes the original concepts of Chinese medicine were significantly modified in their transition to Western cultures. While some experts might dispute some of the authors' conclusions, the book remains a useful insight into Chinese medicine.

The Evidence Base

CHAPTER 12

Clinical research into the effectiveness of acupuncture

Introduction

Acupuncturists need to provide evidence that acupuncture is effective, safe and cost-effective before it can be formally integrated into the policy of any national health service. This does not mean that provision of acupuncture should be forbidden until this evidence is complete and overwhelming – that would risk denying patients a potentially very useful treatment. Individual healthcare practitioners make decisions about using acupuncture or referring patients for treatment on other kinds of evidence: the wishes of the patient, anecdotal reports about the successes of a local practitioner, published case series and audits from local clinics, and the views of their colleagues and opinion leaders. We are currently in a kind of intermediate situation; there is plenty of evidence that acupuncture is likely to be more valuable than other treatments for patients with a particular problem, but not yet enough evidence to convince policymakers to provide it.

Rigorous research into acupuncture is not easy. Acupuncture is a complex intervention, and when considering ways to investigate it we have to think more of the methods used in research into surgery or physical therapy interventions rather than into drugs, particularly the difficulties of blinding the practitioner and the patients. Here, we shall briefly introduce some of the problems in acupuncture research and the ways of interpreting the results of studies with various control groups before summarizing the findings of the research in different conditions.

Blinding participants in acupuncture trials

PROBLEMS WITH 'PLACEBO' ACUPUNCTURE

The gold standard test of a treatment is to compare it with a placebo. There are two reasons for this: (1) to show that the treatment has a *specific* effect (i.e. an effect 'beyond placebo'); only if the treatment is shown to be better than the placebo can we argue convincingly that its effect is not just due to the power of expectation or the therapeutic relationship; and (2) to allow blinding or 'masking' of the patients, so that they are not biased when they are asked to assess the effects of treatment. It is acceptable to use a masked observer instead, to remove bias, but this is may not be possible; for example, pain relies on the patient's verbal report.

A placebo must be indistinguishable from the real treatment, but also inert. Unfortunately, there is no placebo for an acupuncture needle; anything that feels like a needle inevitably has a physiological effect. For many years, researchers have displayed great invention in trying to find inactive controls, but it is now clear that any stimulus on the skin, even pressure or stroking with the blunt end of a needle, can have profound effects on the limbic system when it is being used in a therapeutic context, that is, pretending to be a real treatment (Lundeberg et al., 2009; Pariente et al., 2005). A sharp, penetrating needle has a greater effect than blunt pressure on the skin, but the fact remains that the blunt pressure will have treatment effects of its own through widespread activation of the limbic system; a blunt needle is not an inactive placebo.

> *Stroking or applying pressure on the skin given as 'treatment' has an effect on the limbic system.*

This creates a problem, which is that the effect of the blunt needle is almost as large as the effect of the real needle (Fig. 12.1). The difference between the effects of sharp (penetrating) and blunt (non-penetrating) needles is often much smaller than the difference between a drug and a placebo drug, though a measurable difference seems to be emerging (Vickers, et al., 2012,

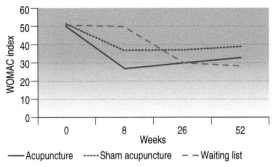

Figure 12.1 Results of a three-armed study showing the response of patients in each arm measured various weeks after the start of the trial; the waiting list group received acupuncture after 8 weeks. The effect of acupuncture is slightly greater than that of placebo, and the difference is statistically significant; both are much more effective than the waiting list. Data taken from an RCT of acupuncture for knee osteoarthritis. *(From Witt, C., Brinkhaus, B., Jena, S., et al., 2005. Acupuncture in patients with osteoarthritis of the knee. Lancet 366, 136–143).*

Vickers et al., 2017). So acupuncture studies that are too small, or not very carefully designed, will fail to reveal this small difference. This is known as a 'type 2 error' – the failure to reveal an effect that does actually exist because of inadequate statistical power.

To avoid misleading readers, we repeat that acupuncture is often very much more effective than other treatments or than no treatment. It is the comparison with blunt needles that is problematic.

'SHAM' ACUPUNCTURE

Since there is no truly inactive 'placebo' control for acupuncture, we should use the term 'sham' instead for any control procedure that aims to make the patient think that they have had treatment. 'Sham' is used for other physical interventions, such as surgery and manipulation. The term 'sham' should be a reminder to us that the control subjects are receiving an intervention which often has some neurophysiological effect.

A 'placebo-controlled', double-blind trial of acupuncture is technically impossible.

There are two types of sham acupuncture: non-penetrating and penetrating sham.

Non-penetrating sham controls

There is almost no limit to the inventiveness of different researchers in trying to achieve a control that does not penetrate the skin. Some have tried tapping the skin with the guide tube, with a cocktail stick or even with a sharpened fingernail; others have designed a special plastic plug at the end of the guide tube so the needle is driven into the plug and prevented from entering the skin. More recently, Streitberger and colleagues (Park et al., 1999; Streitberger and Kleinhenz, 1998) introduced a blunted needle with a loose handle that slides over the shaft rather like a stage dagger. Even these devices have problems: they stimulate the skin sometimes quite strongly, are difficult to conceal reliably, and interfere with the normal needling procedure.

Penetrating sham controls

In many clinical trials, real acupuncture needles have been used in the control group, but in a supposedly incorrect way. The way the needle is used 'incorrectly' determines the actual research question. It can be placed:

- in the wrong site – this tests the effect of putting a needle in the correct place;
- in the right site but only superficially and without stimulation (so-called 'minimal acupuncture') – this tests the effect of deep needle insertion and possibly nerve stimulation;
- both in the wrong site and superficially – this tests the effects of both site and stimulation.

However, it is difficult to find a 'wrong' site that is credible to the patient but does not have some effect on the condition, through segmental analgesia or general regulation. Patients expect to be needled somewhere near the painful problem, but even superficial needling around the area is likely to have some segmental effect. The difference then between the effects of real and sham treatment could be very small indeed.

Needles in the 'wrong' place can still have segmental and general effects.

It may not be easy for practitioners to give a sham treatment, after developing habits of manually stimulating needles ever since they learned acupuncture. In a multicentre study with many practitioners, one might expect sham treatments to be actually quite strongly active.

Technically, it is easy to apply effective acupuncture, but difficult to apply an ineffective sham.

TESTING THE SUCCESS OF PATIENT BLINDING

Blinding should be verified at the end of the trial to make sure the control patients have not realized that they have not been given an active treatment. This is a common criticism of acupuncture studies, and yet another difficulty for designing randomized controlled trials (RCTs) with sham acupuncture.

The best way to test blinding is to ask patients to judge whether they had real or sham acupuncture, but this may interfere with the effectiveness of treatment by unnaturally focusing patients' attention on the treatment. Timing of the question is also difficult: too early and the treatment has not had time to work, too late and the answer will be influenced by the treatment response – so in a study where acupuncture is effective, patients will judge that they have active treatment and the trial will be criticized for failing to ensure blinding!

Verifying patient blinding without interfering with treatment is difficult.

Another solution is to assess how credible the treatment was, using indirect questions such as: 'Would you recommend this treatment to a friend?', or 'Would you expect this treatment to work for another condition you had?' The credibility of the real and the sham treatments can be compared.

PRACTITIONER BLINDING

Ideally, in an RCT the acupuncture practitioner should be blinded (masked) to whether the treatment is real or sham. This is difficult, though not impossible. We know of three ways in which researchers have tried to achieve this.

- A novice was trained specially to give two treatments without being told which was active and which was sham (Lagrue et al., 1977). The lack of skill and experience could reduce the quality of the treatment.
- One acupuncturist examined the patients and devised two treatments for each patient, only one of which was correct (Allen et al., 1998). A second practitioner gave one or the other, according to randomisation. In practice, the treating practitioner might be unblinded.
- A pair of special needles held within tubes was developed, one of which penetrated a section of wadding but not the skin (Takakura et al., 2011). The technicalities would impede normal practice.

For now, we shall have to accept that acupuncturists, like surgeons, cannot readily be blinded in clinical trials. However, participants should be blinded whenever possible and, additionally, the assessors (and those who perform data entry and analysis, ideally) should also be blinded.

Other problems in acupuncture research

CONDITIONS SUITABLE FOR CLINICAL TRIALS

Acupuncture is most commonly used to treat musculoskeletal conditions. It seems particularly effective for these conditions within about 6–12 weeks from the onset (i.e. before they become chronic). However, it is difficult to recruit patients at this intermediate stage, still within primary care and therefore few in number. Recruiting in secondary care risks treating only chronic, less responsive conditions. The results of such trials should not be used as the basis for global statements like 'acupuncture does not work'.

Conditions that respond best to acupuncture are often difficult to research.

Acupuncture research could most profitably concentrate on musculoskeletal injuries, particularly at the stage immediately beyond the time when they might have been expected to heal. Physical therapy settings seem ideal. Other promising conditions include headache, nausea and vomiting, and osteoarthritis of moderate severity.

Lack of research resources: suboptimal acupuncture treatment

Pharmacological research into new drugs follows a well-trodden research pathway: only optimum dosage is tested, and only in ideal patients.

In contrast, many acupuncture trials have been undertaken as one-off studies by enthusiasts. Often treatment is not optimized, for example, by a consensus of expert opinion. For acupuncture studies to have convincing results, we need to know much more about the most appropriate acupuncture for different conditions. We need to undertake preliminary studies comparing different types of acupuncture to find the best for different types of patients – the equivalent of phase I studies in pharmaceutical research.

Lack of knowledge about the optimal acupuncture for different conditions seriously compromises clinical trials.

Often other aspects of acupuncture studies seem to have set them up to fail. Sample sizes have been inadequate, leading to type 2 errors. Treatment has been inadequate. Outcome measures have not been chosen carefully enough, so they are not appropriate and sensitive enough to show subtle effects, and the statistical analysis may not be the most appropriate for the data, perhaps because it cannot deal with baseline differences between the groups.

ACUPUNCTURE AS A COMPLEX INTERVENTION

Acupuncture needles are obviously capable of producing a wide variety of effects, changing over time as they depend to a certain extent on the neurological status of the patient at the time, including anxiety and attitude to acupuncture. This becomes all the more complicated because acupuncture can itself alter the status of the patient – by reducing the anxiety, for example.

RESULTS OF ACUPUNCTURE TRIALS AT ODDS WITH CLINICAL OBSERVATION

The many design problems that we have discussed throughout this chapter all combine to greatly compromise the chance of finding a positive effect of acupuncture. The range of difficulties peculiar to acupuncture research, and the lack of research resources, explains why the results of controlled trials of acupuncture often do not truly reflect the effects that we see every day in practice.

Acupuncturists are convinced of the effectiveness of acupuncture by seeing their patients respond – patients consistently show a reaction that is new to medicine, such as *de qi* sensation, the rapid relief of pain in certain problems such as myofascial trigger points, the pain relief experienced on the following day in other cases of pain, and the side effects such as drowsiness and euphoria. Acupuncturists are convinced of the value of their therapy despite the rather poor trial evidence and feel reassured that better designed studies will produce results that bear out their clinical observations.

> *Acupuncture is highly effective in clinical practice, but its specific effect is difficult to prove.*

In fact, there have recently been some encouraging signs that the quality of acupuncture research is improving, and it is reassuring that many of the newer, more rigorous, better designed studies are producing more convincingly positive results, in conditions as varied as nausea from chemotherapy, to neck pain and chronic knee pain. This in turn is reflected in more positive outcomes of the newer systematic reviews, compared with the older reviews, which were often limited by the poor quality of the studies.

Choice of control group

The control group must be chosen to address the intended research question. The control groups most commonly used are:

- *No additional treatment, for example, patients on a waiting list:* the question here is whether acupuncture is better than the treatment that patients are already using, such as drugs. Acupuncture has shown itself superior to usual care for many conditions, often by a considerable margin. This may be partly expectation, but the results indicate the effects we might see with acupuncture in practice.
- *Another treatment:* the comparison with other available treatment options is relevant in making decisions about care. The only way to show a treatment's specific effect, over and above expectation, the clinical setting, or the therapeutic interaction, is a placebo-controlled trial.
- *Sham acupuncture:* given the practical difficulties of 'placebo acupuncture' discussed earlier, it is likely that sham-controlled studies are unreliable and false-negative results are highly likely. Large, very carefully designed trials are needed.
- *Other placebos:* a few studies have used other placebos as a control – placebo tablets, placebo TENS and so on. However, these are likely to have different psychological impacts from acupuncture.

Landmarks in acupuncture clinical research

THE GERMAN INSURANCE COMPANY STUDIES

Several German health insurance companies sponsored a series of rigorous studies to inform their decision whether to reimburse acupuncture treatment. They ran the studies in patients with headache (tension headache or migraine), neck pain, back pain, and knee and hip osteoarthritis.

As well as large, observational studies to measure the overall safety and effectiveness of acupuncture, they sponsored large RCTs comparing acupuncture with usual care, and smaller, three-arm RCTs comparing acupuncture both with sham acupuncture and with waiting list or superficial needling in 'incorrect' locations (Cummings, 2009; Linde et al., 2006; Witt et al., 2006a).

To summarize these results:

- there were large overall treatment effects and a high level of safety,
- acupuncture was at least equivalent to standard care (for migraine), or much better than standard care (chronic low back pain, knee osteoarthritis),
- the effectiveness of acupuncture in RCTs was the same as in everyday practice,
- acupuncture generally showed at least a trend towards being superior to sham acupuncture but only reached statistical significance for knee pain. (Bear in mind that sham acupuncture in these studies was likely to be an active treatment.)

On the strength of these results, the insurance organizations decided to provide funding for acupuncture treatment of two conditions:

1. Osteoarthritis of the knee – because it is better than sham acupuncture, and the effect size is useful.
2. Back pain – because, although acupuncture was not proven to be better than sham acupuncture, low back pain is an economic disaster for which the standard care has little to offer; therefore, it is sufficient that acupuncture proved to be better than standard care.

INDIVIDUAL PATIENT DATA META-ANALYSIS (IPDMA)

The most reliable evidence comes from combining the individual patient's results from the best RCTs. Vickers and colleagues combined 29 studies on four chronic pain conditions: back and neck pain, osteoarthritis, chronic headache, and shoulder pain (Vickers et al., 2012). There was a total of 17 922 participants. As shown in Table 12.1, acupuncture was superior to both sham and no-acupuncture control for each pain condition ($P < 0.001$ for all comparisons).

Results were expressed as 'effect size'. In round figures, the effect size of acupuncture against sham is 0.2 (small size) and against usual care is 0.5 (medium size) in these painful conditions. The authors gave an example of what these effect sizes mean in real terms: a baseline pain score on a 0–100 scale for a typical RCT might be 60. Given a standard deviation of 25, follow-up

TABLE 12.1 ■ Effect sizes in 29 studies (Vickers et al., 2012)

Pain location	vs Sham	vs no-acupuncture control
Spine	8, 0.37 (0.27, 0.46)	7, 0.55 (0.51, 0.58)
Osteoarthritis	5, 0.26 (0.17, 0.34)	6, 0.57 (0.50, 0.64)
Chronic headache	4, 0.15 (0.07, 0.24)	5, 0.42 (0.37, 0.46)
Shoulder pain	3, 0.62 (0.46, 0.77)	0

(Reproduced with permission from Filshie, J., White, A., Cummings, M. (Eds) Medical Acupuncture: A Western Scientific Approach. (Second edition) Elsevier, Edinburgh. 2016. p. 308.)

scores might be 43 in a no-acupuncture group, 35 in a sham group and 30 in patients receiving traditional acupuncture.

Effect sizes of 0.2 are regarded as small, 0.5 as medium and 0.8 as large.

This study provides the most distinct evidence to date that acupuncture is more than just a placebo. The overall effect of acupuncture (specific and non-specific), as experienced by patients in routine clinical practice, is clinically relevant.

NETWORK META-ANALYSIS

If treatment A and treatment B were compared with control C in different studies, a network meta-analysis combines the results to compare the treatments with each other. Corbett and colleagues compared all studies of all physical treatments used for the pain of knee osteoarthritis (Corbett et al., 2013). Acupuncture proved to be the most effective treatment of all, (see Table 12.2) and this result was confirmed when using the results of the best 42 RCTs.

Assessing the evidence

We shall now summarize the evidence for a range of conditions in which acupuncture may be helpful, mainly using systematic reviews. We are not presenting an all-inclusive review of the evidence here; for example, we do not consider the laboratory studies in humans, of which there are many. This chapter is intended as an introduction to the strengths and weaknesses of the evidence base of acupuncture. We believe that the evidence here can be thought of as a pointer to the main areas in which acupuncture is most likely to be fully integrated into Western medical care.

We shall consider the evidence about the cost-effectiveness of acupuncture in a separate section towards the end of this chapter.

Acupuncture for musculoskeletal conditions

NECK PAIN

Neck pain is a condition which, according to many practitioners' clinical experience, seems to respond more quickly and satisfactorily than almost any other.

TABLE 12.2 ■ **Effect sizes of various physical treatments of knee osteoarthritis pain**

Intervention	Studies, effect size (95% CI)
Acupuncture	24, 0.89 (CI 0.59, 1.18)
Balneotherapy	9, 0.65 (CI 0.15, 1.04)
TENS	12, 0.65 (CI 0.25, 1.06)
Aerobic exercise	11, 0.55 (CI 0.21, 0.89)
Sham acupuncture	14, 0.47 (CI 0.09, 0.84)
Muscle-strengthening exercise	28, 0.40 (CI 0.19, 0.61)
Weight loss	5, 0.26 (CI −0.15, 0.67)
No intervention	5, −0.44 (CI −1.04, 0.15)

(Reproduced with permission from Filshie, J., White, A., Cummings, M. (Eds) Medical Acupuncture: A Western Scientific Approach. (Second edition) Elsevier, Edinburgh. 2016. p. 309.)

The large German RCT on neck pain ($N = 14\,161$ total cohort; $N = 3766$ randomized) clearly demonstrated the effectiveness of acupuncture compared with usual care (Witt et al., 2006a). The economic analysis that formed part of this study found the cost per additional QAL Y of acupuncture in chronic neck pain was €12 469.

The individual patient data meta-analysis found an effect size (SMD) of 0.8 for neck pain (contrasting with SMD 0.2 for back pain). That seems to fit our clinical impression that neck pain responds more often and probably reflects the higher proportion of muscular pain elements in neck pain presentations. (Vickers et al., 2012)

In primary care, patients usually present with acute or subacute neck pain. There are no RCTs specifically on this group, but evidence from primary care shows that patients respond quickly and satisfactorily (Ross et al., 1999).

UPPER LIMB PAIN

The research into acupuncture for shoulder pain is dominated by two huge studies.

Molsberger and colleagues gave either acupuncture, sham acupuncture or usual physical therapy to 424 outpatients with chronic shoulder pain (Molsberger et al., 2010). The acupuncture was given to tender points and classical points around the shoulder, as well as leg points such as ST38 or GB34. After 3 months, pain scores were halved in 65% of the acupuncture group, 24% of the sham acupuncture group and 37% of the standard therapy group. These differences were significant ($P < .01$).

The second RCT of shoulder pain included 425 patients with chronic symptoms of unilateral subacromial syndrome (rotator cuff tendinitis or subacromial bursitis, in some cases associated with capsulitis) (Vas et al., 2008). Fifteen sessions of physiotherapy were given during the 3 weeks that the treatment lasted and were randomized to additionally receive, once a week, acupuncture or mock TENS (transcutaneous electrical nerve stimulation). Acupuncture was given deeply to the single point ST38, with four stimulations in a period of 20 minutes. It is important to note that the painful shoulder was mobilized during needle stimulation or mock TENS, and the patients went straight into an hour of physiotherapy immediately afterwards. The acupuncture group had better scores at the end of treatment and at 12 months: 34% of the acupuncture group recorded pain compared with 71% of the sham-TENS and exercise group.

Tennis elbow (lateral epicondylitis) often responds in clinical practice so could be a good candidate for research, and it is surprising that there are few studies of high quality (Tang et al., 2015). Two studies were positive. In the first ($N = 82$), Haker and colleagues found deep needling at acupuncture points was more effective than superficial needling at the same points (Haker and Lundeberg, 1990). In a second study ($N = 55$), Fink and colleagues found 10 treatments (twice per week) with genuine acupuncture were superior to needling at inappropriate sites, when the patients were assessed 2 weeks after the end of treatment (Fink et al., 2002).

Low back pain

A systematic review found 31 studies of acupuncture for low back pain (Yuan et al., 2015). Combining ten sham-controlled RCTs in chronic low back pain showed a significant effect on pain up to 3 months after treatment, though because of differences between studies the result is not highly reliable. No effect on disability was found, interestingly, and the comparison with medication showed only a trend. The individual patient data meta-analysis (discussed previously) found an effect size (SMD) of 0.2 compared with sham, and an SMD of 0.5 against no acupuncture controls. (Vickers et al., 2012)

An RCT in primary care in the United Kingdom ($N = 239$) compared acupuncture with usual care alone. Acupuncture was superior for one of the measurements of pain, showing a trend at

12 months and a significant difference at 24 months (Thomas et al., 2005). However, there was no difference between the groups in the assessment of impairment of function using the Oswestry score.

Overall, then, acupuncture has a role to play in managing chronic back pain. Its success rate may not be too impressive but is quite respectable in comparison with other treatments. The German insurance companies decided to reimburse acupuncture for back pain for that very reason.

LOW BACK AND PELVIC PAIN IN PREGNANCY

In one study of 60 women, acupuncture was superior to physiotherapy in relieving pain and disability (Wedenberg et al., 2000). Another study, in Gothenburg, involved 386 pregnant women with pelvic girdle pain (PGP), who all received standard treatment (Elden et al., 2005). Women who received acupuncture in addition had significantly reduced pain, and acupuncture was also superior to specific stabilizing exercises.

A Cochrane review of eight studies (1305 participants) of physical interventions found acupuncture and stabilizing exercises relieved PGP more than usual prenatal care, and acupuncture provided more relief from evening pain than exercise (Liddle and Pennick, 2015), similar to the results of a second review (Ee et al., 2008). The research is promising but limited, and further studies are planned (Foster et al., 2016).

CHRONIC KNEE PAIN

In a systematic review of 13 RCTs (involving 2362 patients) of acupuncture for chronic knee pain, mainly due to osteoarthritis (White et al., 2007), the authors set five criteria for 'adequate' acupuncture:

- at least six treatments
- at least once per week
- at least four points needled
- for at least 20 minutes
- either manual stimulation to elicit *de qi* or electrical stimulation of sufficient intensity to produce more than minimal sensation.

In addition, they specified that sham controls could only be called 'true sham' if they avoided needling in the legs in the same segments as the knee joint. A meta-analysis of five trials with adequate acupuncture showed that acupuncture was clearly superior to sham acupuncture for both pain and function, both in the short term and over a period of 6–12 months (see Fig. 12.2).

The results are robust and are supported by the five higher quality studies included in the IPDMA (Vickers et al., 2012). Effect sizes were 0.26 against sham and 0.57 against no acupuncture. A subsequent review of 10 studies found significant short-term effects for pain and short- and long-term effects for function (Lin et al., 2016a).

A network meta-analysis showed acupuncture to be more effective than other conservative treatments for knee pain, including exercise (Corbett et al., 2013).

In view of these advantages and acupuncture's high level of safety, acupuncture should clearly be considered a genuine alternative to (the usual) non-steroidal anti-inflammatory drugs for chronic knee pain, with their known long-term effects. Yet some official guidelines, including those of the National Institute for Health and Clinical Excellence, still decline to recommend it.

MYOFASCIAL PAIN

In clinical practice, certain types of myofascial pain, after injury for example, respond most rapidly to acupuncture and are one of the most satisfying conditions to treat. We might, therefore, expect

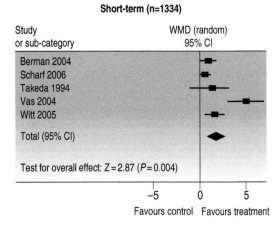

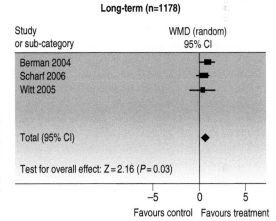

Figure 12.2 Results of meta-analyses of short-term and long-term effects of acupuncture on chronic knee pain. Subsequent studies have not shown any substantial difference. *(From White, A., Foster, N.E., Cummings, M., et al., 2007. Acupuncture treatment for chronic knee pain: a systematic review. Rheumatology (Oxford) 46 (3), 384–390.)*

to find plenty of research into it. A review noted inconsistencies in making the diagnosis (Tough et al., 2007). Early reviews found too few studies to give a consistent picture, but the 16 studies accumulated in a review (Wang et al., 2017) gave a consistent picture of significant pain relief from eight sessions, sometimes fewer.

FIBROMYALGIA

Fibromyalgia should be clearly distinguished from myofascial trigger point pain, most obviously by the fact that myofascial trigger point pain is generally unilateral and has relatively few psychological consequences. Fibromyalgia is diagnosed by the presence of pain above and below the waist and on both sides of the body for at least 3 months, with tenderness to pressure at 11 of 18 defined points. Ninety-six per cent of patients with fibromyalgia also have fatigue and 86% have insomnia (Wolfe et al., 1990).

The RCTs of acupuncture for fibromyalgia have mixed results, which may reflect some doubt about the best approach to treatment, as patients with fibromyalgia may be unusually responsive to treatment or can be easily made worse. A review of 16 RCTs found acupuncture superior to conventional medication in reducing pain scores but not superior to sham acupuncture (Cao et al., 2013). It seems that acupuncture may be helpful for some individuals with fibromyalgia but not others.

OTHER MUSCULOSKELETAL CONDITIONS

There are few trials on acupuncture for osteoarthritis (OA) of the hip, but the large pragmatic study from the German insurance company series found that the effects of acupuncture on hip pain were similar to the effects on knee pain (Witt et al., 2006b). There is not enough evidence from RCTs to draw any useful conclusions about the role of acupuncture in treating inflammatory arthritis, such as ankylosing spondylitis or rheumatoid arthritis.

Acupuncture for headache

MIGRAINE

The majority of studies on migraine have investigated the role of acupuncture in prevention, that is, treatment given in between attacks. A Cochrane review included 22 RCTs (4985 participants) with at least 8 weeks' duration (Linde et al., 2016a). Acupuncture was superior to no acupuncture in reducing headache frequency, with an effect size of 0.56; frequency of migraine episodes halved in 41% of patients who received acupuncture and only 17% of controls. Acupuncture was also slightly, but significantly, superior to sham acupuncture for headache frequency and at least as good as medication for several outcomes.

The question whether acupuncture has any value in the treatment of *acute* migraine was studied in one trial ($N = 179$), which compared acupuncture with injection of sumatriptan and with a sham injection (Melchart et al., 2003). If given in the early stages, acupuncture and sumatriptan both blocked the development of full-blown migraine in 35% of patients, whereas sham did so in only 18%. However, if the first treatment failed and the headache became established, then sumatriptan was more effective than acupuncture. Acupuncture caused significantly fewer side effects than sumatriptan.

TENSION-TYPE HEADACHE

Chronic tension headache – defined as headache that occurs more than 15 days a month – is an almost intractable condition and a hard test for acupuncture. Headaches that occur on less than 15 days a month (classified as episodic tension headaches) do respond to some interventions, including acupuncture. In some patients tension headache symptoms may be closely linked to TrPs in the shoulders and neck, and it may be these patients who respond best to treatment.

A Cochrane review of acupuncture in tension headache found 12 RCTs: over 40% of patients responded to acupuncture with a halving of headaches, compared with less than 20% in the no acupuncture groups (Linde et al., 2016b). As with migraine, acupuncture was slightly but significantly superior to sham acupuncture (see Fig. 12.3).

Acupuncture for respiratory conditions

ALLERGIC RHINITIS

The evidence from RCTs is fairly consistent that acupuncture provides both prevention and acute relief of symptoms in allergic rhinitis. A review combining all available 13 studies, whatever the control intervention, found acupuncture effective for symptom scores, medication use and quality-of-life scores (Feng et al., 2015). In one high-quality study with 422 patients, acupuncture was

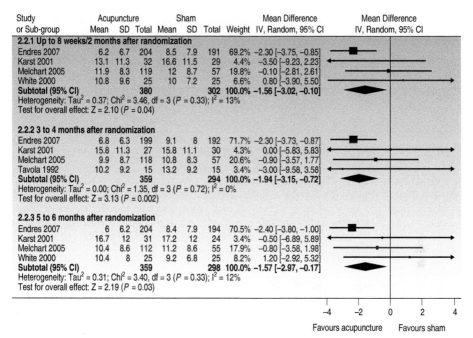

Figure 12.3 Results of meta-analyses of acupuncture compared with sham interventions for tension-type headache, showing the effect on number of headache days at various times after the course of acupuncture (*From Linde, K., Allais, G., Brinkhaus, B., et al., 2016b. Acupuncture for the prevention of tension-type headache, in: Linde, K. (Ed.), Cochrane Database of Systematic Reviews. John Wiley & Sons, Ltd, Chichester, UK CD007587. Reproduced with permission.*)

superior to sham acupuncture and relief medication alone for (seasonal) allergic rhinitis (Brinkhaus et al., 2013). The effect was still noticeable in the following year's allergy season. However, the treatment is probably not cost-effective within the public health system.

Acupuncture for addictions

There is a considerable amount of basic research into the mechanisms of dependence, and a great deal of interest in the influence that acupuncture may have on these mechanisms. Demonstrating any effects clinically is notoriously difficult because of differing settings, lack of certainty about optimal treatments, and high levels of dropout in this population.

The overall result of a systematic review of RCTs of acupuncture for smoking cessation found it (slightly) superior to sham acupuncture, but there were features that made the evidence unconvincing (White et al., 2014). However, a subgroup of studies that used continuous stimulation in the ear, whether with an indwelling needle or a pressure device, found them superior to sham interventions, at least in the short term.

Seven studies of acupuncture for alcohol dependence were included in a systematic review which concluded that acupuncture was more effective than various control interventions for reducing alcohol-related symptoms and behaviours (Shin et al., 2017).

Evidence into any role of acupuncture in cocaine and opioid dependence is inconclusive. Future research may usefully concentrate on the relaxing and motivating effects of acupuncture in rehabilitation settings (Chang et al., 2010) rather than relapse rates.

Acupuncture for central nervous system conditions

There is a great deal of laboratory research that suggests various mechanisms by which acupuncture, particularly EA, may assist recovery from stroke, including by improving reperfusion, by increasing neuronal plasticity and by neuroprotection. However, the clinical research at the time of writing has not shown any convincing clinical benefit from the treatments used so far.

One area where acupuncture might prove to have value is in spinal cord injury, for which a systematic review found improvement in functional scores and in bladder dysfunction (Heo et al., 2013).

Acupuncture for nausea and vomiting

Acupuncture treatment for nausea and vomiting is relatively easy to research, since patients are plentiful and effects are short-term, so they are easy to monitor. The standard treatment usually applied is simply PC6 bilaterally, but in clinical practice ST36 and possibly abdominal points are used – therefore many studies might have used inadequate treatment. Other studies used acupressure or electrical stimulation.

NAUSEA OF PREGNANCY

Because of risks to the foetus from medication, acupuncture is commonly considered during pregnancy. Early studies suggested a powerful effect but were criticized for being poorly controlled.

A careful review of 29 studies published in English or Chinese, using a variety of treatment techniques and settings, found no convincing evidence that acupuncture or acupressure have an effect that is clinically useful (Van den Heuvel et al., 2015).

POSTOPERATIVE NAUSEA AND VOMITING

A review of 59 RCTs ($N = 7667$ participants) found acupuncture for postoperative nausea and vomiting significantly reduced nausea scores and use of medication compared with sham acupuncture (Lee et al., 2015). The evidence overall is only moderate quality, but two very rigorous studies showed positive results. Acupuncture is as effective as anti-emetic medication.

NAUSEA AND VOMITING FROM CHEMOTHERAPY

A review of 11 trials ($N = 1247$) found that acupuncture reduced the proportion of patients with nausea or vomiting (Garcia et al., 2013). Most trials were at risk of bias except one, which found EA superior to sham (minimal) needling and to standard medication for high-dose chemotherapy (Shen et al., 2000). Episodes of vomiting were reduced from 15 (with medication) to 5 (with EA) over 5 days. Clinical guidelines specifically recommend acupressure and acupuncture (Greenlee et al., 2017).

Acupuncture for genitourinary and reproductive medicine

GYNAECOLOGICAL CONDITIONS

For dysmenorrhoea, a review found inconsistent evidence: acupuncture was not superior to sham but was superior to anti-inflammatory analgesic drugs (Smith et al., 2016)

There are now a number of studies that suggest that acupuncture has a useful effect on postmenopausal hot flushes. A large observational study has also shown a prolonged valuable effect of acupuncture, including self-acupuncture, on hot flushes in cancer patients (Filshie et al., 2005). However, the effect has not been shown to be superior to sham acupuncture (Dodin et al., 2013), and the review suggested that the evidence is not all of reliable quality.

INFERTILITY

In the area of infertility, the research so far suggests that acupuncture may have a number of beneficial actions, though the evidence is not conclusive, possibly because of the variety of treatments and timing schedules and settings (Carr, 2015a). There is evidence that low-frequency EA to the abdominal muscles (with or without stimulation to points in the legs) increases uterine blood flow (Stener-Victorin and Humaidan, 2006), which may improve uterine function before embryo implantation in in-vitro fertilization (IVF). Treatment given during the follicular phase as well as around embryo transfer appears more successful than a single treatment (Carr, 2015a).

POLYCYSTIC OVARY SYNDROME

Controlled trials find acupuncture effective at reducing amenorrhoea and inducing ovulation, and the success rate increases with more intense treatment (Stener-Victorin, 2016).

ACUPUNCTURE IN PREGNANCY

The effects of acupuncture on pelvic pain and back pain and on nausea in pregnancy are reviewed in the relevant sections of this chapter.

Acupuncture seems to be useful in reducing pain in labour and increasing satisfaction according to a review (Smith et al., 2011). A large observational study of nearly 18 000 women found that the patients who chose acupuncture during labour were less likely to require epidural analgesia (Nesheim and Kinge, 2006). There is also some evidence that acupuncture ripens the cervix at term and shortens labour (Smith, 2016).

Urological conditions

A conventional medical intervention, posterior tibial nerve stimulation (PTNS), is clearly derived from EA treatment to SP6 unilaterally and is recommended for overactive bladder symptoms. EA itself is probably adequate (Pullman, 2016). An RCT in 39 women showed that acupuncture is as effective as treatment with the standard anticholinergic drug oxybutinin, with significantly fewer adverse events and, as a result, significantly fewer dropouts from the study (Kelleher et al., 1994).

A review of seven RCTs found acupuncture superior to sham acupuncture and to medication in the treatment of chronic prostatis/chronic pelvic pain syndrome (Qin et al., 2016).

The cost-effectiveness of acupuncture

Several reports show cost savings after introducing acupuncture into practice, from reduced prescriptions (Myers, 1991) and reduced referrals (Lindall, 1999; Ross, 2001).

Rigorous evaluation of the economic aspects of treatments depends on careful measurement of the actual cost of treatment in relation to the improvement in patients' health. The patients' health is assessed by a standard measure called the QALY (quality adjusted life year), which takes into account both the prolongation of life (if any) in years and the quality of life during that

TABLE 12.3 ■ The cost-effectiveness of acupuncture, from full economic evaluations of randomized controlled trials

Condition (first author)	N =	Context	Cost per quality adjusted life year
Back pain (Ratcliffe et al., 2006)	241	Private acupuncturist	£4241
Low back pain (Witt et al., 2006c)[a]	2388	Physician acupuncturist	€10 526
Headache (Wonderling et al., 2004)	401	Private physiotherapist	£9180
Headache (Witt et al., 2008a)[a]	2682	Physician acupuncturist	€11 657
Neck pain (Willich et al., 2006)[a]	3005	Physician acupuncturist	€12 469
Osteoarthritis knee or hip (Reinhold et al., 2008)[a]	421	Physician acupuncturist	€17 845
Dysmenorrhoea (Witt et al., 2008b)[a]	201	Physician acupuncturist	€3011
Allergic rhinitis (Witt, 2009)[a]	981	Physician acupuncturist	€22 798
Allergic rhinitis (Reinhold, 2013)[a]	364	Physician acupuncturist	€20 807–€74 585

Original costs reported.
[a]Conducted in Germany. Other studies conducted in the UK.
(From Kim, S. Y. et al., 2012. A systematic review of cost-effectiveness analyses alongside randomised controlled trials of acupuncture. Acupunct Med 30, 273–85.)

time, on a scale of zero (dead) to one (in complete health). This measure operates in the same way for all treatments in all conditions and, thus, allows a true comparison of the cost-effectiveness of different treatments. Now, acupuncture does not extend life in any condition (except, arguably, in smoking cessation), so its effects are measured solely by the increase in quality of life after treatment. When acupuncture is compared with usual care, the comparison is known as the 'ICER' (incremental cost effectiveness ratio); this measures the cost of improving the patients' health with acupuncture. The units are '£ per QALY'.

In the United Kingdom, The National Institute for Health and Clinical Excellence (NICE) uses ICERs to evaluate the place of new treatments, and as a general rule will recommend treatments that cost less than £20 000 per QALY.

The economic analyses of acupuncture included in a definitive review (Kim et al., 2012) are summarized in Table 12.3. With the exception of treatment of allergic rhinitis, these estimates are competitive compared with many accepted medical interventions.

The main cost of an acupuncture service is the cost of the acupuncturist, including the overheads, such as professional development and management of the service. In reality, resourceful practitioners will find ways of reducing these costs to a minimum in order to be able to provide a valuable service to their patients. Many practitioners already employed in the health service incorporate acupuncture into their everyday practice without diminishing the care of other patients. Others treat several patients at the same time, in groups (Berkovitz et al., 2008; White et al., 2012). This kind of arrangement can significantly improve the cost-effectiveness of acupuncture and is well worth investigating as a means of delivering acupuncture effectively in a resource-limited health service.

Summary

Clinical research into the effectiveness of acupuncture is confounded by the lack of a reliable placebo form of acupuncture, which leads to corresponding difficulties blinding patients, blinding practitioners, and measuring effects rigorously; other problems are difficulties in recruiting patients in the conditions in which acupuncture is most effective, lack of information on the optimal treatment for many conditions, and choice of control group.

Landmarks in acupuncture research include a series of insurance company–funded studies in Germany, an individual patient-data meta-analysis (Vickers et al., 2012), and a network analysis (Corbett et al., 2013).

In musculoskeletal conditions, acupuncture has been convincingly shown to be superior to sham treatments for chronic knee pain, and the best evidence is positive for treating neck pain, low back pain and upper limb pain. It is also cost-effective for some of these conditions. Migraine and tension-type headaches now join the list of conditions for which the evidence is positive on balance, as do nausea and vomiting from various causes, especially postoperative and chemotherapy-induced.

A form of treatment clearly derived from electroacupuncture, viz posterior tibial nerve stimulation (PTNS), is effective for overactive bladder symptoms.

Evidence on the safety of acupuncture

Introduction: acupuncture is safe in skilled hands

Acupuncture has a reputation for safety, and this has now been confirmed by a number of large prospective surveys in different countries.

In one survey between 1998 and 2000, 78 doctors and physiotherapists in the United Kingdom reported adverse events that occurred during or after 32 000 consultations involving acupuncture (White et al., 2001). No serious adverse events were reported, and minor events, such as bleeding, occurred on average in less than 7% of treatments. These figures are essentially similar to the findings of other studies among trained practitioners and in a variety of countries, such as a survey of 34 000 treatments by 1848 non-medical acupuncturists over a 4-week period in the United Kingdom (MacPherson et al., 2001); a survey of over 65 000 treatments given in a Japanese acupuncture clinic, which found nothing more serious to report than nine cases in which a needle was not removed at the end of treatment (Yamashita et al., 1999); and a survey of 3535 acupuncture treatments by 29 doctors and other health professionals in Germany (Ernst et al., 2003).

Finally, 13 579 German physicians recorded adverse events on 229 230 patients, each receiving an average of 10 acupuncture treatments – approximately 2.2 million sessions (Witt et al., 2009). The overall AE rate was 8.6%, over half of which were bleeding; 2.2% of patients experienced an event that required some form of treatment from the practitioner – mostly, pressure to stop bleeding. Two patients suffered pneumothorax, one of whom required hospital admission. The longest lasting event – 180 days – was a nerve injury in the lower limb. AEs that indicated any degree of negligence amounted to 0.1% of the total.

Acupuncture is used at various locations in the British National Health Service (NHS), and like all treatments, it is monitored by reporting of adverse events to a national register. In a 2-year period, there were 3.7 million patient safety reports, 325 involving acupuncture (Wheway et al., 2012). Patients found needles left in place after treatment (59 cases); patients were 'forgotten' in a cubicle and treated longer than intended (41 cases); and patients experienced dizziness or faintness without loss of consciousness (99) and with temporary loss of consciousness (63). Eight patients fell off the couch during or immediately after treatment, and four fell down outside the clinic, after treatment. There were seven incidents of bruising or soreness at the needle site and one incident of a small blister. There were five possible incidents of pneumothorax of which two were confirmed diagnoses; one was classified as 'severe'. The authors commented that acupuncture 'seems to be a low harm treatment'. However, there is clearly room for improving the administrative aspect of treatment.

An editorial in the *British Medical Journal* that reviewed the evidence from these various surveys summarized the situation thus: 'Acupuncture ... certainly seems, in skilled hands, one of the safer forms of medical intervention' (Vincent, 2001).

One of the strengths of the safety record of acupuncture is that, since it is mainly used to treat musculoskeletal pain, it is replacing drugs such as non-steroidal anti-inflammatory drugs (NSAIDs). These have several major side effects, particularly upper-gastrointestinal bleeding or perforation, increasing the risk of this by a factor of about four (Hernandez-Diaz and Rodriguez, 2000), as well as causing renal damage, hypertension and increased risk of stroke and myocardial infarction (Bally et al., 2017).

The evidence on safety of acupuncture is not as straightforward as it may appear from the overall picture given by the surveys, however. Their results showed that there is wide variation in the rate of adverse events reported by different practitioners. For example, one practitioner reported bleeding in 53% of patients after acupuncture, whereas others reported no bleeding at all. Some of this variation will be due to differences in reporting – practitioners who tend to be very cautious are likely to report every small bleeding event, even though the survey's intention was to record only significant amounts of bleeding. Also, some of the variation between individual practitioners may be due to differences between their types of patients (e.g. a practice consisting of elderly patients might expect more bleeding because they may have more fragile vessels and less subcutaneous tissue), and some may be due to different styles of acupuncture. But it also seems likely that adverse events do vary with the technique and skill of the practitioner.

Practitioners should not simply think 'acupuncture is safe', but be alert to reducing adverse events as much as possible.

Detailed recommendations for the safe practice of acupuncture are given in Chapter 16, and in this chapter we are concentrating solely on a discussion of the published evidence. Knowing what has happened before helps us to avoid doing the same.

Apart from problems from the needling, there is another potential source of risk to patients from acupuncture: they may miss out on conventional treatment that would have been more effective for their condition. This so-called 'indirect' risk can obviously be serious, for example, if patients are not given the chance of an early diagnosis of their cancer because their symptoms are not interpreted correctly. This book is written with the assumption that every patient considered for acupuncture will have undergone a conventional medical diagnosis and will have been informed when conventional treatment would give a better likelihood of recovery than acupuncture can offer.

Wise men learn by other men's mistakes; fools learn from their own. (Anon)

The potential risks of acupuncture

It is useful to discuss adverse events in three degrees of severity, as shown in Table 13.1.

It is not easy to obtain reliable figures about the rates of risk in acupuncture, because there are inevitably biases and inaccuracies in reporting. Adverse events may be underreported by patients because they do not want to upset their practitioner; they are underreported by the acupuncturist who may not be aware of the ethical need to describe such events, but overreported by other health professionals who dislike acupuncture for some reason and wish to damage its reputation.

TABLE 13.1 ■ A classification of mild, significant and serious adverse events, as used in this chapter

Severity	Definition
Mild	Reversible, short-lived and does not seriously inconvenience the patient ·
Significant	Needs medical attention or interferes with the patient's normal activities
Serious	Requires hospital admission or prolongation of existing hospital stay, or results in persistent or significant disability/incapacity or death

Also, *attribution* of any event to acupuncture treatment may not be straightforward. It may be difficult to know whether an event was caused by acupuncture or not. There are standard methods of attributing cause, including the time relationship of onset and offset, biomedical rationale, and repeated sequelae on reexposure. However, in individual cases, especially the more serious and complex ones, several events may contribute to the outcome, and the precise contribution of different causes cannot be accurately deduced.

The figures for the rates of adverse events given here are based on the published evidence but should be regarded as only an approximation. Anyway, our main interest is practical, so learning how we can make acupuncture practice safer is a major objective in this book.

MILD EVENTS

The most common events during or after acupuncture, with typical incidence rates (expressed as a per cent of treatments, reported by practitioners (White, 2006), are:
- bleeding, more than a small drop of blood: about 3%
- aggravation of symptoms: about 1–2%
- needling pain, more than a little sharpness: about 1%
- drowsiness: up to about 1%
- faintness: usually less than 0.5%

This rate of minor adverse events is low enough to be officially classed as 'minimal'. Other events that are less commonly reported include nausea and headache.

Two minor events – aggravation of symptoms and drowsiness – need further comment. Some practitioners argue that acupuncture is a 'natural' treatment, it is inevitable that it will make problems worse before they improve, and any aggravation of symptoms is an acceptable part of 'the healing response'. This idea may reassure patients, but there is no evidence that it is true. In one study in which the incidence of aggravation was recorded together with the eventual outcome, aggravation was not followed by a better response to treatment; the rate of success in patients is about 70%, with or without aggravation. Plenty of patients respond to treatment without getting worse first. This all suggests that aggravation may not, in fact, be necessary for a response to acupuncture, and we, therefore, recommend that practitioners should take care to avoid aggravation, particularly by not using too strong a treatment at the first session.

Relaxation is often regarded as a benefit of treatment, but drowsiness can be serious enough to increase the danger posed by anyone who is driving or using machinery. In one study, about one-third of patients experienced some degree of drowsiness (Brattberg, 1986), and only slightly less experienced drowsiness in a recent study (MacPherson and Thomas, 2005).

SIGNIFICANT EVENTS

Skin infections that need treatment have been reported on a number of occasions. These generally involve the typical opportunistic commensal bacteria, but four cases of infection with *Mycobacterium* have been reported. Cases of cellulitis have occurred when acupuncture needles were inserted into areas of oedema. Occasionally, acupuncture seems to reactivate herpes infection.

Peripheral nerve injury from acupuncture has been reported on a few occasions leading to, for example, foot drop. The question arises as to why this kind of nerve injury is not reported more often when acupuncture needles must penetrate nerves quite frequently? The usual explanation given is that acupuncture needles have non-cutting tips, which push the nerve fibres apart.

Exacerbation of asthma is not uncommon during or after treatment and may be serious enough to require hospital admission.

Seizures can occur in patients who faint because they are treated sitting up (which is not recommended, for this reason). Very occasionally, a seizure occurs in a patient who is lying down. Here the diagnosis may be reflex anoxic seizure due to a marked vagal response to needling, involving the limbic system.

Other kinds of major collapse during acupuncture are rare, but some have been reported. A few patients have been reported to simply go unconscious, either when the needles are inserted or when they are stimulated. There is no associated cardiovascular collapse, so the mechanism must be purely neurological. If not already supine, such patients need to be laid down immediately. Fortunately it is extremely rare, and the patients recover completely.

SERIOUS EVENTS

These are very rare and are either traumatic or infectious.

Trauma is usually caused by needling too deeply or in the wrong place, and sometimes by the patient moving either spontaneously or during muscle stimulation by EA.

Pneumothorax is the commonest serious adverse event of acupuncture (Xu et al., 2013) and has caused several deaths. It can be caused by needling either the anterior or posterior chest wall. Symptoms can arise immediately during treatment or may develop gradually over the following 48 hours.

There is little room for error in depth of needling for thin, emaciated patients, though there is also a risk in needling overweight or obese patients as it can be difficult to judge the actual depth of a needle in relation to the thicker tissue layers.

Injury to the *central nervous system* is next most commonly reported (Xu et al., 2013), including penetration of the medulla and intracranial bleeds – from needling sites in the neck. The peripheral nervous system is open to injury, for example, peroneal, median and facial nerves.

Cardiac tamponade can develop with catastrophic speed, and various other injuries to heart muscle and blood vessels have also been reported (Xu et al., 2013).

Infections may be local or systemic. The most serious local infections are those that develop into necrotizing fasciitis, with 20%–30% mortality rate. Deaths have been reported (White, 2004). The source of infection may be the practitioner. Many cases of *Mycobacterium* skin infection were reported at clinics in Korea; in one clinic, they were traced to improper sterilization of towels and packs placed on acupuncture points after the needles were withdrawn, and in another clinic to improper preparation of the fluid used to clean the skin (Xu et al., 2013).

Systemic infections have changed pattern since single use disposable needles were introduced. Hepatitis from contaminated needles used to be common and is still a problem in certain countries (Nguyen et al., 2007). *Staphylococcal* infection is now more common, and methicillin-resistant varieties have been reported (Xu et al., 2013).

Serious adverse events can be almost completely eliminated by good practice.

The overall risk of serious adverse events associated with acupuncture was estimated from the evidence of 13 prospective studies involving over 4 million treatments that reported 11 events, none of which were fatal (White, 2006). The cumulative worldwide rate for serious adverse events with acupuncture is, therefore, estimated to be 0.02 per 10000 treatments, which represents 'negligible' risk, well below that of most medical treatments.

Overall, acupuncture presents a 'negligible' risk of adverse events.

Unavoidable events

There is no doubt that some reactions to acupuncture are unavoidable in that they are inevitable in individual patients but cannot be predicted. These reactions are described in every survey, even those of Japanese acupuncture in which needles are generally inserted very superficially into the subcutaneous layer only. The most serious of these is severe drowsiness, which may constitute a real risk of road traffic accidents. Clearly some patients are more susceptible than others. The decision on whether to give acupuncture to such patients again depends on a risk–benefit assessment: the same reaction is likely to recur on further treatment, though drowsiness is one reaction that generally becomes less severe when the treatment is repeated.

Drowsiness after acupuncture can be serious; patients must be advised how to manage it.

Indirect risk

The risk from acupuncture is described as 'indirect' if the harm is caused by the practitioner rather than the practice. This would usually be when a patient does not receive more appropriate treatment because the practitioner made an incorrect diagnosis or believed acupuncture to be more effective than it is in this case or was not aware of the evidence that acupuncture is less effective than other treatment.

Summary

Acupuncture is generally safe in skilled hands, as shown by the evidence from several prospective surveys. One of acupuncture's strengths is its safety compared with other treatments.

Acupuncture does carry some risks and can be a source of 'indirect' risk if it is used instead of another more effective treatment. The rates of adverse events vary from practitioner to practitioner, and each has a responsibility to develop and maintain safe practice. The most common mild adverse events after acupuncture are bleeding, pain on needling and aggravation of symptoms, followed by faintness and drowsiness (which may affect driving). Significant events are less common and include skin infections, peripheral nerve injury, exacerbations of asthma and seizure. Serious events are very rare. Some side effects are unavoidable. Overall, the risk of adverse events from acupuncture is 'negligible'.

Practical Aspects

Preparation for treatment

Introduction

Acupuncture is in some senses a straightforward matter of inserting a few needles, but for treatment to be safe and effective, some preparation is necessary. It is particularly important for beginners to establish good habits and routines as soon as they start practice. Safety, just as much as effectiveness, must become second nature when treating patients.

As well as ensuring that they have the best training and continued education, acupuncturists should apply the standards expected of all healthcare professionals; they should conduct themselves at all times in a suitable manner, as directed by their professional body or regulator.

One aspect of good patient care is that there is appropriate communication between all the practitioners involved in the patient's care. Acupuncturists who work independently should try to ensure (with the patient's permission) that the patient's general practitioner knows that they are seeing the patient, for both clinical and for ethical reasons.

Practitioners must have a realistic and honest approach to what the acupuncture can achieve. Claims that acupuncture can treat anything and everything are false, deceive patients, and bring the therapy into disrepute. Acupuncture is a form of therapy with successes and failures, like most treatments.

This chapter describes the thinking processes behind safe and effective acupuncture, up to the moment of inserting the needles. The treatment itself is described in Chapter 15. This chapter has not been designed to be used as the basis for formal guidelines for providing services, and readers who need to develop guidelines could base them on an example written for palliative care (Filshie and Hester, 2006).

Patients suitable for acupuncture

We do not recommend treating minors, at least before gaining considerable experience in handling both children and needles, as many adverse events have been reported (Vohra et al., 2011).

All patients considering acupuncture should be screened for possible contraindications and for the need for special precautions.

CONTRAINDICATIONS

The patient must be willing to receive acupuncture. There are two main reasons why the patient might not be willing:
1. Needle phobia
2. Personal belief: occasionally, patients believe that acupuncture, because it is associated with ideas of energy and meridians, can have an adverse spiritual influence, so they want nothing to do with it. It is tempting to try to circumvent these beliefs by using some phrase like 'dry needling', but probably not sensible. We prefer to mention the word 'acupuncture' and let the patient decide.

A tiny proportion of the population can react to an invasive medical technique by having a convulsion; the mechanism is not clear, but may involve a sudden strong vagal stimulus to the heart. The significance of this reaction is that it cannot necessarily be avoided by treatment with the patient lying flat. This should not be confused with the sort of mild anoxic convulsion that can occur if a patient faints and cannot immediately be lain down flat. If there is a history of an unexplained convulsion in a patient presenting for acupuncture, it is wise to avoid acupuncture treatment. Inevitably, acupuncture treatment might be the first time this reaction appears, in which case such events should be regarded as unavoidable.

Patients who bruise spontaneously should not be treated until their clotting function has been checked and is satisfactory.

These contraindications are listed in Box 14.1.

ABSOLUTE CONTRAINDICATIONS TO PARTICULAR TECHNIQUES

Indwelling needles are a potential source for bacteraemia, which can infect a damaged heart causing subacute bacterial endocarditis. (High risk: previous endocarditis, previous cardiac surgery, including valve prosthesis and congenital valvular disease, such as Marfan's syndrome; low risk: rheumatic heart disease, calcified aortic valve and floppy mitral valve.)

Electrical stimulation may possibly affect the sensing mechanism of a pacemaker or intracardiac defibrillator.

RELATIVE CONTRAINDICATIONS: BALANCING RISK AND BENEFIT

A patient may have a 'relative' contraindication to acupuncture. In this case it is the practitioner's responsibility to work with the patient in striking a balance between the benefits and risks of treatment. For example, faced with a patient who has a bleeding disorder due to anticoagulant drugs, you may decide not to use deep needling for treating ankylosing spondylitis. The expectation

---

Box 14.1 ■ Contraindications for acupuncture

Absolute contraindications to acupuncture

- Patient unwilling
- Spontaneous bleeding or bruising (until fully assessed)

Absolute contraindications to a particular technique

- Valvular heart disease: avoid indwelling needles
- Demand-type pacemaker or intracardiac defibrillator: avoid electroacupuncture across the chest

Relative contraindications

- Severe bleeding tendency, for example, anticoagulant therapy, thrombocytopenia
- Psychologically disturbed patients (may have unpredictable reactions)
- Compromised immune system
- Previous seizure induced by an invasive medical procedure
- Marked previous reaction to acupuncture

Box 14.2 ■ Cases where special precautions are required in using acupuncture

Special precautions

- Bleeding tendency (see text)
- Epilepsy: do not leave the patient unattended
- Immunosuppression, whether due to medical condition or drug treatment: extra attention to hygiene
- Pregnancy (see text)
- Patients without a clear diagnosis: acupuncture may mask symptoms of serious conditions, such as cancer, delaying diagnosis
- Abnormal physical structure: increased risk of trauma, especially if underweight
- Patient who needs to drive after acupuncture treatment: treat lightly, rest and observe after treatment and advise to stop driving if drowsy
- Strong reactors to acupuncture (see text)
- Patients with peripheral neuropathy: avoid areas of neuropathy

---

of benefit is small, and deep needling runs a significant risk of causing haemorrhage. On the other hand, you might use superficial needling to treat tension headaches, as it is safe and could be effective. Take the patient's views into account, but do not allow a patient to persuade you to give treatment when you believe it is contraindicated.

SPECIAL PRECAUTIONS

This section deals with precautions that can be anticipated from the condition of the patient (Box 14.2). There are additional precautions that are necessary due to local conditions at the point, which will be discussed in Chapter 15.

PATIENTS WITH A BLEEDING TENDENCY

A bleeding tendency due to conditions such as haemophilia, thrombocytopenia, or taking anti-coagulant drugs is a 'relative contraindication', but if you decide to treat the patient then you

---

Box 14.3 ■ Acupuncture used in a patient with thrombocytopenia

A 39-year-old woman developed thrombocytopenia in her second pregnancy. She had a caesarean section under general anaesthetic, since spinal and epidural anaesthesia were contraindicated by her platelet count of 82×10^9/l. In the postoperative phase, standard analgesic drugs did not provide sufficient pain relief, but acupuncture had a rapid, useful effect, without causing excessive bleeding (Oomman et al., 2005).

---

should take special precautions. It might be hard to justify needling patients who have extremely low platelet counts, for example, but acupuncture may be a useful alternative for patients with moderate bleeding disorder (Box 14.3).

In patients with a bleeding tendency, acupuncture should be performed with particular care:
- Consider using fine needles, perhaps with electrical stimulation for the less sensitive patients.
- Avoid deep or vigorous needling in the enclosed fascial compartments of the lower limbs and forearms because of the potential risk of compartment syndrome.
- Take particular care when needling near joints because of the increased risk of haemarthrosis.
- Apply firm pressure to points after removing the needles.

PREGNANCY

Many acupuncture teachers advise their students to use acupuncture carefully, if at all, in the first trimester of pregnancy on the grounds that 'it may cause a spontaneous abortion'. However, even at full term there is little evidence that acupuncture can induce labour. Acupuncture is frequently used in China to treat many conditions in the first trimester of pregnancy without applying any special precautions. Its use in early pregnancy is also clearly established in the West for treating nausea.

Acupuncturists who are nervous of litigation will argue: 'Even if you don't cause an abortion, you may be blamed if one occurs within a few days of your acupuncture session'. This is defensive medicine, which often does not lead to good treatment. There is good evidence from large observational studies and 15 controlled trials that the outcomes of pregnancy (both pregnancy outcomes and health of child) are not affected by acupuncture (Carr, 2015b)). We suggest that:
- acupuncture can be used throughout pregnancy;
- risks and benefits of treatment are weighed in the usual way;
- in the first trimester, it is probably wise to avoid strong stimulation techniques.

STRONG REACTORS

Some patients react strongly to acupuncture. When given normal strength treatment, they are more than usually likely to experience:
- aggravation of their symptoms;
- feelings of fatigue immediately after treatment;
- feelings of malaise after treatment, sometimes amounting to an influenza-like syndrome for 2 or 3 days.

About 5–10% of a primary care population will have a reaction to a dose of treatment that has no adverse effect on the remaining 90–95%, but the rate is higher in cancer patients.

It is difficult to judge a patient's sensitivity in advance. Felix Mann observed that artistic types and those who have a strongly charitable outlook are more likely to be strong reactors. Sometimes a patient will give a clue in that a previous physical treatment – massage or manipulation, for example – produced an unpleasant reaction. In that case it is best to assume that acupuncture will do the same.

Fortunately, strong *reactors* are also usually good *responders*. These patients have a strong therapeutic response, so treatment can be light; in the most sensitive patients, as little as 30 seconds' needling may be enough.

Similarly, children in general are likely to be strong reactors and the needle should be removed within a few seconds. However, unlike adults, this does not mean that all children are good responders.

PATIENTS WITH CANCER

Acupuncture can be very helpful for the palliation of symptoms in cancer patients, but special precautions are required for many reasons, including the facts that these patients may have significant side effects of their treatment and even multiorgan disease. There is a risk of masking symptoms, and a need to recognize that a patient who fails to respond to treatment in the usual way may have an increased tumour load. A fuller discussion of these issues is available for anyone who wishes to treat these patients (Filshie, 2001).

ANXIOUS PATIENTS

Acupuncture is likely to be more effective in patients who are not anxious during treatment because of the effects of raised CCK release (Chapter 9). Patients should have their questions and anxieties addressed during preparation for treatment.

Information and informed consent

Patients must be given adequate information about the benefits and risks of acupuncture to allow them to make a fully informed decision about treatment. The difficulty is in knowing what is meant by 'adequate' information, but it should include an offer of:
- realistic information about the possible expected benefits of acupuncture,
- information about the known risks of acupuncture relevant to the case,
- other available treatments for the condition, if relevant.

It is obviously important to strike a balance between, on the one hand, not concealing risks that are real and relevant and, on the other hand, officiously listing every adverse event that has ever been associated with acupuncture. This could frighten patients away from using a treatment that might benefit them.

All information about risk must be given in plain language that is appropriate for the individual patient, and you should judge (and ideally justify) when individual patients have gained the information they need and want. Patients should also be offered information about the risks and benefits of any other treatment available. It would be unethical to recommend acupuncture for a condition when there is no convincing evidence that it is effective, when some other treatment is known to be effective. Patients must be informed and then make their own decision.

Normally, verbal consent to treatment is enough. Some hospital trusts or other employers of acupuncturists may insist on providing written information and sometimes obtaining signed consent. The patient information leaflet reproduced here (Box 14.4) was developed by consent between several UK acupuncture professional organizations. It includes an optional space for patient consent, but a signature is less important, legally speaking, than making sure that patients are satisfied that they have enough information to make a decision. Practitioners who wish to use the form in their own practice may download it from http://www.medical-acupuncture.co.uk/journal/2001(2)/page_123.pdf.

In fact, patients are considered to have given consent *for the examination* by preparing themselves, that is, by undressing or by climbing on the couch, after being given adequate information. It

---

Box 14.4 ■ Patient information sheet and consent form

Please read this information carefully and ask your practitioner if there is anything that you do not understand.

What is acupuncture?

Acupuncture is a form of therapy in which fine needles are inserted into specific points on the body.

Is acupuncture safe?

Acupuncture is generally very safe. Serious side effects are very rare – less than one per 10 000 treatments.

Does acupuncture have side effects?

You need to be aware that:
- drowsiness occurs after treatment in a small number of patients, and, if affected, you are advised not to drive,
- minor bleeding or bruising occurs after acupuncture in about 3% of treatments,
- pain during treatment occurs in about 1% of treatments,
- symptoms can get worse after treatment (less than 3% of patients). You should tell your acupuncturist about this, but it is usually a good sign,
- fainting can occur in certain patients, particularly at the first treatment.

In addition, if there are particular risks that apply in your case, your practitioner will discuss these with you.

Is there anything your practitioner needs to know?

Apart from the usual medical details, it is important that you let your practitioner know:
- if you have ever experienced a fit, faint or funny turn,
- if you have a pacemaker or any other electrical implants,
- if you have a bleeding disorder,
- if you are taking anticoagulants or any other medication,
- if you have damaged heart valves or any other particular risk of infection.

Single-use, sterile, disposable needles are used in the clinic.

Statement of consent

I confirm that I have read and understood the above information, and I consent to having acupuncture treatment. I understand that I can refuse treatment at any time.

Signature

Print name in full

Date

---

might be natural to assume that this consent includes having treatment, but be aware that further consent may be needed because:

- patients may be willing to be examined but want to reserve the right to decide on treatment after the examination;
- you may not be able to predict the possible benefits of treatment until you have examined the patient, in which case you should provide this information then.

Also, if you have been using manual acupuncture and want to introduce electroacupuncture, it is worth discussing this with the patient if electroacupuncture was not expressly included in your initial discussion about acupuncture.

Conditions suitable for acupuncture

Acupuncture is most often used for various musculoskeletal problems (Table 14.1). Myofascial trigger point pain seems to respond quickest and best, followed by other soft-tissue injuries

TABLE 14.1 ■ **Some common conditions for which patients request acupuncture, and a general indication of the likelihood of a useful clinical response**

Response likely	Response possible: moderate or limited cases	Response unlikely: rare or idiosyncratic
Musculoskeletal conditions		
Trigger point pain (myofascial)	Fibromyalgia	Disease process, in inflammatory
Osteoarthritis (especially knee, ankle, acromio-clavicular joint, cervical spine)	Postlaminectomy syndromes Shoulder pain	arthropathies, including ankylosing spondylitis
Lateral and medial epicondylitis		
Neck pain[a]		
Unilateral back pain		
Other knee, calf and foot pains; condition labelled as Morton's metatarsalgia		
Other painful conditions		
Tension-type headache	Chronic widespread non-specific back pain[a]	Tinnitus
Atypical facial pain		Motor spasm after stroke
Dental pain, with no obvious treatable dental cause	Painful diabetic neuropathy, other painful peripheral	Epilepsy Multiple sclerosis symptoms
Non-cardiac chest pain	neuropathies	Parkinson's
Trochanteric bursitis, condition		
Neurological		
Migraine	Spinal pain related to nerve root entrapment or impingement	
	Neuropathic pain or pain from true neuromas	
	Complex regional pain syndrome	
	Ischaemic pain	
	Phantom limb pain	
	Raynaud's disease	
	Neurogenic pain (e.g. trigeminal neuralgia)	
	Central ('thalamic') pain	
Abdominal conditions		
Dysmenorrhoea	Symptoms of ulcerative colitis or Crohn's disease, irritable	Bladder outlet obstruction
Irritable bowel syndrome presenting mainly as pain	Bowel syndrome presenting mainly as disturbance of bowel function	Generalized or systemic skin conditions (e.g. psoriasis)
	Urinary incontinence	
Conditions without pain		
Nausea		
Hay fever, allergic rhinitis		
Xerostomia, dry eyes		
Menopausal hot flushes		
Reversible local skin conditions		

[a]Symptoms and signs of neurological involvement make a response less likely. This table is based on clinical experience, case series and randomized controlled trial evidence, and, therefore, includes the possible benefits of the effects of the expectation associated with acupuncture.

that have been slow to heal, followed by osteoarthritis. Acupuncturists disagree among themselves about which conditions respond best, because their opinions are formed by anecdotes of particular patients they remember doing well or badly, and because a practitioners' particular interest in a condition might improve their skill and influence their approach and raise expectations.

Acupuncture will not reverse structural changes, like the degeneration of joint surfaces in osteoarthritis, though it can still give symptom relief and reduce inflammation. This fact may be obvious to the practitioner but should be made explicit to the patient who may misunderstand what friends have told them and may come for acupuncture believing, for example, that it will heal their arthritic joints.

The patient's history may suggest that the symptoms could be due either to underlying pathology or to myofascial trigger points (MTrPs) imitating the condition. It may be difficult to be sure clinically, since MTrPs could be present in both cases. Patients respond to acupuncture better when the symptoms are caused primarily by trigger points. For example, dysmenorrhoea due to endometriosis is less likely to be helped much by acupuncture, but similar symptoms from trigger points in the abdominal wall are more likely to respond.

Nociceptive pain responds more reliably than neuropathic pain or pain of no known cause, and acupuncture for these conditions should be regarded as a kind of therapeutic trial.

Like many other therapies, acupuncture works best on earlier and milder cases, before the disease pattern becomes thoroughly ingrained and complicated with psychological changes.

If the expectations of both the patient and the practitioner are positive, then success seems more likely – though acupuncture can certainly be effective in patients who seem to have very low expectations of it helping. It is important for practitioners' expectations for acupuncture to be realistic and to make sure that patients who have unrealistic ones can be gently disabused without having their hopes completely dashed.

Acupuncture equipment

STANDARD NEEDLES

Acupuncture needles consist of a shaft and a handle. The shaft is generally stainless steel, sometimes coated in silicone, and handles may be of metals or plastic, as shown in Plate 1. The various features of the needles are listed in Table 14.2.

There have been reports that silicone fragments may break off the surface coating and (theoretically) provoke foreign body reactions, but this is a risk common to all silicone-coated hypodermic needles and surgical instruments, not just acupuncture needles.

TABLE 14.2 ■ Variations in needle manufacture

Part	Variations	Advantages/disadvantages
Shaft (stainless steel)	Unpolished	Standard: 'gripped' by the tissues to produce *de qi*
	Polished	Patient comfort, but less grip on tissues so *de qi* may be more difficult to elicit
Handle	Wound metal (steel, copper)	Easy to manipulate
	Solid metal	Less easy to manipulate
	Plastic	Lightweight[a] but non-conductive

[a]In some positions, a needle that is lying superficially will be more likely to fall out if the handle is heavy steel, in which case lightweight plastic can be an advantage.

Needles vary in quality. Badly manufactured needles may have loose metal fragments that can become detached or have hooked tips (Xie et al., 2014).

The needle tip does not simply taper to a point like a pencil, but has a rounded profile (traditionally likened to a pine cone), as shown in Fig. 14.1. This is supposed to be less traumatic – pushing tissue fibres apart rather cutting them – but it can still damage blood vessels, nerves and other structures if the needle or the patient moves. The modern needle is manufactured to a high standard, but occasionally the point is blunt or hooked or the handle not firmly attached to the shaft. Such needles should be rejected as soon as the problem is discovered.

The typical diameter and length (which refers to the exposed part of the shaft, not including the handle) of acupuncture needles commonly used are shown in Table 14.3.

Only purchase single-use disposable needles.

GUIDE TUBES

Traditionally, needles were inserted directly using a deft flick-and-twist action, but now most needles are available with plastic guide tubes, and these are recommended for beginners. The needle is about 2 mm longer than the tube, enough to allow it to be inserted through the skin by tapping the end. Single needles are usually held in the guide tube with a wedge or plug. After freeing the needle, tip the guide tube so the handle appears and hold it between finger and thumb to stop it from falling out.

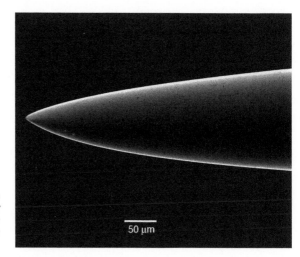

Figure 14.1 Electronmicrograph of an acupuncture needle tip. *(Courtesy of Dr Roy Moate, Plymouth Electron Microscopy Centre, Plymouth University.)*

50 µm

TABLE 14.3 ■ **Variations in dimensions of needles commonly available**

	Range	Standard	Special purposes
Diameter	0.12–0.35 mm	0.25 or 0.30 mm	Longer needles should be thicker, for strength; typically 0.30 or 0.35 mm
Length	7–125 mm	25 or 40 mm	Longer lengths up to 75 mm are used for deep points (e.g. in the gluteal muscles) Shorter lengths, 15 mm, are used in the face and ear

OTHER TYPES OF NEEDLE

Indwelling needles are sometimes used to continue the effect of treatment between attendances at clinics. There are special contraindications and precautions for using them, which we discuss in Chapter 17. The most common form of indwelling needle is like a tiny drawing pin with a 2 mm projection (Plate 9). They are made in various diameters and sometimes have an integral adhesive dressing (Fig. 14.2). They are sometimes used for auricular acupuncture (when they may be called 'press studs'), but we discuss the potential dangers of this in Chapter 17. They may also be used at other sites and need to be fixed securely with an adhesive dressing (Plate 10).

Auricular acupressure can be applied using stainless steel balls or, more traditionally, seeds of the *Vaccaria* plant, as shown in Plate 11.

ELECTROACUPUNCTURE EQUIPMENT

While some practitioners never use electroacupuncture (EA) in the whole course of their professional career and, presumably, their patients are pleased with the results, most find that, before long, they want to be able to use EA particularly for patients with chronic pain.

Choosing EA equipment is not straightforward. Cheap stimulators are available that are sometimes effective, but apparatus that is really flexible and reliable enough costs several hundred pounds. It is worth buying the best you can afford. Some of the most important criteria for a quality machine are suggested in Box 14.5. Some of the older models that are still available do not perform as described and might not meet current standard quality criteria; in Europe, standards

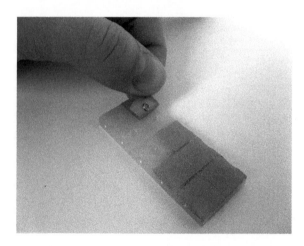

Figure 14.2 Photograph of indwelling needle with integral adhesive dressing.

Box 14.5 ■ Suggested features of optimal electroacupuncture apparatus

- low-voltage operation, preferably battery-powered
- master on/off switch
- square wave output with waves of alternating polarity
- low- intermediate- and high-frequency outputs (e.g. 2–4 Hz, 10–15 Hz, and 80–100 Hz), with automatic switching between them
- separate adjustment for the intensities of low-frequency and high-frequency outputs
- at least three pairs of output leads, each with its own intensity control
- each intensity control placed in line with its output socket, for easy identification

are set by the International Electrotechnical Committee (CEI), but there are, as yet, no specific standards for EA machines. An example of currently available apparatus is shown in Plate 2; it has a maximum current of about 20 mA, which produces about one-sixth the maximum transthoracic electrical charge recommended by the US Food and Drug Administration (John Thompson, personal communication). Some employers insist that all new equipment should be checked by a hospital physics department or similar laboratory.

ANCILLARY EQUIPMENT

It is essential to have these items close at hand when treating patients:
- facilities to wash and dry the hands before treating each patient (alcohol gel is an acceptable alternative),
- couch and pillows to support the patient in the correct position,
- cotton wool swabs to press on the point after removing the needle,
- safe disposal boxes for used needles and swabs,
- facilities for keeping records.

Practitioners who use a separate side room for acupuncture, so they can leave patients relaxing during treatment, should have an intercom or call system for the patient and a method of reminding themselves that there is a patient in the examination room.

RESTERILIZING NEEDLES

In certain circumstances where it is impossible to use single-use disposable acupuncture needles for one reason or another, the only way to deliver acupuncture may be to reuse needles after sterilizing them. Full, hospital-standard sterilization is absolutely essential to avoid transferring infection, for example, hepatitis virus between patients. Needles rapidly become blunt when repeatedly heated up during the sterilization process and are then painful for patients.

The setting for acupuncture

Now that health clinics and hospitals in the West routinely meet high standards, it is easy to forget the relevance of the treatment setting to safe practice. In two cases reported in the literature, patients who were severely debilitated by chronic illness were given acupuncture at their own home and developed septicaemia, which ultimately contributed to their death. Their condition suggests their immune systems were compromised, but unhygienic conditions probably contributed to the septicaemia.

The setting for acupuncture practice must offer certain facilities:
- for adequate examination: good light and good access,
- for adequate treatment: anatomical landmarks must be identifiable (e.g. to establish the surface anatomy of the pleura); patient adequately supported on a firm surface so depth of insertion can be monitored (sometimes difficult in the patient's home, which constitutes a real hazard).

Other aspects of the setting that are relevant for safety include having adequate *time* to carefully conduct the procedure and having sufficient *active support* from other staff and colleagues.

Preparation of the practitioner

This is a checklist of items that practitioners should reflect on before starting treatment to ensure that they:
- have the knowledge and skill – both in medicine and in acupuncture – to treat the patient safely and appropriately,

- have formed (or been informed of) a diagnosis and treatment plan,
- in collaboration with the patient, have determined that the potential benefits of using acupuncture in this patient's circumstances outweigh the risks,
- have considered the possible effects of acupuncture on any other condition present,
- have checked that the setting and equipment are satisfactory,
- know the anatomical relationships of all the points they plan to treat,
- can cope with all likely adverse events that might arise,
- have indemnity insurance in place.

Finally, practitioners should ensure their hepatitis B immunization is up to date, not only to protect themselves but also to protect their patients. One small cluster of hepatitis B infections was attributed to spread from the practitioner who was himself antigen positive. This virus is highly infectious in minute doses.

Summary

This chapter is the first of three that are essential reading before using acupuncture in clinical practice. It describes and lists the conditions that must be present for you to make the decision to use acupuncture.

Acupuncture is contraindicated absolutely if the patient has a needle phobia or is not willing and if the patient bruises spontaneously and has not had their clotting function checked. There are a number of relative contraindications. Particular acupuncture techniques are also contraindicated in certain situations.

Special precautions need to be taken for particular patients, such as those with bleeding disorders, epilepsy, or immunosuppression. Particular care should be taken in pregnancy (which is not a contraindication), patients without a clear diagnosis, with any distorted anatomy, and strong reactors. Patients must give their informed consent to treatment, which depends on being given adequate information tailored to their needs and abilities to understand. Consent is generally implied by the fact that patients make themselves ready for treatment, but signed consent may be required in particular circumstances.

Acupuncture should be used for appropriate conditions, and nociceptive pain generally responds better than neurogenic pain.

Acupuncturists should ensure they have good quality basic acupuncture and other equipment and facilities, and an appropriate setting.

CHAPTER 15

Effective needling techniques

CONTENTS

Introduction

Do not start reading the book here! This chapter discusses the basic needling techniques for effective practice. It assumes that you have read Chapter 14, completed the preparatory checks, and understood the Western medical approach to acupuncture. Also, it is essential to read Chapter 16 on safety before starting practice, since safety is of equal importance to effectiveness.

Readers will be familiar by now with our suggestions for the 'standard' doses of treatment to activate the different mechanisms. This chapter describes a standard technique in more detail and the ways in which the dose can be adjusted for the individual patient. This adjustment has to be judged for each patient individually according to the responses – both the immediate response to the needle stimulation and the effects that they experience over the next few hours and days, in both their symptoms and their general well-being. This chapter is about getting the dose of acupuncture right, though the best tutor should be your own reflective clinical practice.

The methods of varying the dose of acupuncture (the strength of treatment) are mainly based on clinical experience rather than systematic research. As readers will expect, we do not consider all the finer variations in treatment that are described in books of traditional Chinese medicine but cover what we believe to be reasonable according to current understanding. You will not, for example, find details about whether to rotate the needle clockwise or anticlockwise, but you will find a discussion of the strength of stimulation.

Dose of acupuncture

Effective treatment with acupuncture means choosing the point or points for this condition in this patient and then needling them with a dose that achieves the right response without causing an adverse reaction. Our general recommendation is to start with a standard treatment in case

TABLE 15.1 ▪ **Factors involved in the strength of sensory stimulation that may affect the dose of an acupuncture treatment**

Treatment variable	Range
Type of point	Myofascial trigger points (MTrPs) are 'strongly effective' when very active (painful) and relevant to the presenting complaint; for other points, the major classical points such as LI4 are strongest, followed by classical points, and local non-traditional points are weakest
Number of points	Minimum treatment involves one point only; usual treatment involves between 4 and 10 points
Needle type	Larger diameter may have greater effect; highly polished surface reduces effect
Number of needle insertions	Each insertion counts separately
Depth of insertion	Increasing strength from superficial to muscular and then to periosteal levels
Needle stimulation	Increasing from none, to manual once, manual several times, and finally to electrical stimulation
Responses elicited	Amount of *de qi*, twitch response of muscle, or muscle contraction with electroacupuncture
Needle retention time	Longer is generally considered to be stronger, up to about 30 minutes maximum
Treatment frequency	Usually weekly, or twice weekly, but may be up to 5x per week
Total number of treatments	Typical courses are about six sessions, but sometimes long-term intermittent 'top-up' treatments are necessary to maintain relief

the patient is sensitive, even if you anticipate that more needles with greater stimulation and longer retention will be needed; it is better to gradually increase the dose, once you know how the patient reacts. The treatment variables are shown in Table 15.1.

Simple ways to reduce the dose of treatment are:
- use thinner needles
- use fewer needles
- insert the needles superficially
- reduce the amount of needle stimulation
- reduce the time the needle is retained.

Acupuncture: basic technique

Standard manual acupuncture, that is, the insertion of a needle into the tissues usually with some form of stimulation, is the most commonly used form of acupuncture throughout the world. The aim is to produce an adequate stimulation in the safest and least painful way. We describe the process in five phases:

1. Insert the needle through skin.
2. Advance the needle to the required depth, usually in a perpendicular direction.
3. Manipulate the needle, if required and if appropriate (considering patient and condition).
4. Retain the needle in situ, if required.
5. Remove the needle.

No needle should be inserted without preparation (Chapter 14) and without considering safety (Chapter 16) including, for example, the posture of the patient and the practitioner's anatomical knowledge.

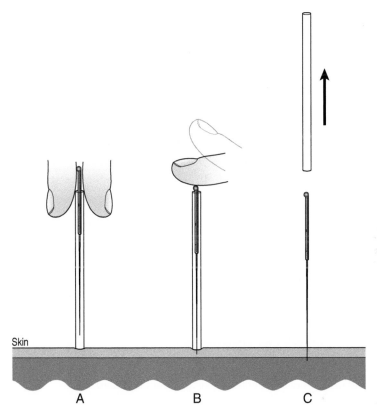

Figure 15.1 Diagram indicating that the needle can be held securely in the guide tube if it is slightly retracted, and that a smart tap with the finger tip will insert the needle subcutaneously, allowing the guide tube to be carefully lifted away.

INSERTION

This should be swift and painless; use the guide tube supplied with needles and tap the needle handle with confidence (Fig. 15.1). Tell patients that they will feel the tap, but they probably will not notice anything sharp – though they may do so occasionally, particularly if the skin is hot and sweaty. If there is a sharp pain, then the needle has hit a nerve, or a richly innervated vessel wall or fascial layer. Try adjusting the needle first, either a little deeper or move superficial, but if the pain does not settle then remove it. If the pain continues even after removing the needle, one of the best ways to stop it is to swiftly reinsert the needle close to the site. This usually stops the pain, but you need to be confident in your actions.

Establish the habit of counting the number of needles inserted (*and* their guide tubes), preferably twice, and recording the number in an orderly way so you can check later that you have taken all the needles out – again counting twice to help avoid human error.

ADVANCE

Once inserted, the needle is situated in the subcutaneous tissue; it will hang sideways if not supported, and it can be left there for 'superficial' needling. But it needs to penetrate deeper either to elicit *de qi* or to inactivate a trigger point. Most acupuncture points are situated over muscle, and a few over loose connective tissue (e.g. BL60 and KI3, just anterior to the Achilles tendon). Usually, therefore, the needle is advanced into the muscle layer, and slight resistance can be felt as it passes through the fascia.

The direction of advancement is usually perpendicular to the skin; important exceptions are when needling over the rib cage and sternum (see the next section).

MANIPULATION

The needle can be manipulated with two techniques, illustrated in Figure 3.3:

1. 'Lift and thrust', that is, repeated vertical movements of about 1–2 cm. (This is also known as 'sparrow pecking'.)
2. Rotation – rapid rotation about 90° in alternate directions using index finger and thumb.

Do this until the patient feels *de qi*. Often, at about the same time, the tissues grip the needle. The components of *de qi* are described in Chapter 4; most practitioners do not tell patients exactly what to expect so as not to bias their description of the sensations.

The individual needling response is quite variable, though we do not understand why, and there are some patients in whom it is difficult or impossible to achieve *de qi* at all. If you cannot elicit *de qi* in a patient for whom you think it is necessary, reinsert the needle a few millimetres away and try again. But more than two or possibly three insertions at one location are enough for any patient.

The technique for inactivating MTrPs is slightly different and is described in the section called Needling myofascial trigger points, below.

If any manipulation becomes unpleasantly painful or aversive, stop.

Please note that some practitioners choose not to manipulate the needles at all once they have been inserted to their desired depths (including one of the editors!).

RETENTION

There is a long tradition in acupuncture treatment of leaving patients lying quietly with their needles in situ for about 20 minutes ('needle retention'), which tallies with the time taken for CSF β-endorphin concentrations to reach their maximum levels. Needles are usually left for this time for segmental, extrasegmental and central effects. However, good responses may be obtained after 10 minutes. Treatment of MTrPs does not need to be prolonged, and clinically many cases with tender points other than trigger points seem to respond to a few minutes' needling, perhaps through the axon reflex (see Chapter 5). Patients can relax deeply in about 10 minutes, but 20–30 minutes lying down is even more likely to result in relaxation or sedation if you have the facilities to allow this.

REMOVAL

Usually each needle can be pulled straight out; many practitioners then press briefly on the point with a cotton wool ball (not a finger – you could spread infection, such as hepatitis), to stem any tiny spot of bleeding. Sometimes needles become bent by muscle contraction, which may be due to electroacupuncture (EA) or the patient's own movement. Bent needles have to be coaxed out more carefully. Very occasionally a needle breaks accidentally, and if it could cause damage to particularly vital structures (e.g. pleura, spinal cord, eye), then it could constitute a surgical emergency. The needle must be removed in any event under imaging, unless the tip is visible to the naked eye when buried in soft tissue.

Finally, check that all the needles have been removed and safely placed in a sharps container.

Guide tubes should also be accounted for, since patients or cleaners may be unfamiliar with the apparatus and may regard them as dangerous.

Count the needles in, twice; count the needles out, twice.

Acupuncture: variations on the basic technique

NEEDLING MYOFASCIAL TRIGGER POINTS

If the myofascial trigger point (MTrP) is acutely tender and the pain is intense (signs of a highly active MTrP), then needle it cautiously.

In normal cases, fix the MTrP with one finger on either side of, or along, the band and advance the needle onto the MTrP, keeping eyes and fingers ready to identify a twitch response. This has been shown to predict a good response, as does a reproduction of the patient's pain (Hong et al., 1997). Often the MTrP will not be found the first time, or several MTrPs will be present in one muscle; in both cases it will be necessary to readvance the needle at a slightly different angle, exploring the muscle in a fan-like pattern (Fig. 15.2) – but avoid withdrawing it completely from the body to save having to reinsert it through the skin. When no more twitches can be produced, withdraw the needle and press the area to prevent bleeding within the muscle, as this causes posttreatment soreness.

Choose a needle that is long enough to reach the MTrP; for example, piriformis cannot be reached with the standard 30 mm needle and needs one of at least 70 mm.

SUPERFICIAL NEEDLING

In Japan, particularly for non-painful conditions, needles are usually inserted into the points subcutaneously, without stimulation. This technique is also used by many practitioners in the West, and called 'minimal' or 'superficial' acupuncture (Baldry, 1993; Mann, 1992). In Japan the needles are retained for 20 minutes or so, but in the West practitioners who use superficial acupuncture generally state that as little as half a minute may be enough to produce treatment effects. Baldry described this as a useful method of de-activating trigger points.

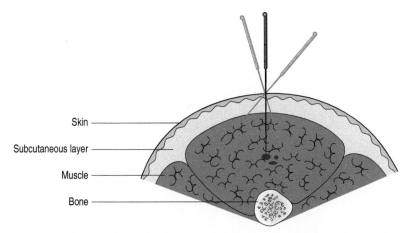

Skin
Subcutaneous layer
Muscle
Bone

Figure 15.2 Diagram illustrating in principle how to explore fanwise with a needle to eliminate all parts of a myofascial trigger point. The needle is withdrawn only as far as the subcutaneous layer, so that it does not need to be reinserted through the skin.

PERIOSTEAL PECKING AND STRONG STIMULATION

In contrast to superficial needling, a strong treatment has evolved in the West. It is called 'periosteal pecking' and involves choosing a point where the bone is readily within reach of the needle (usually around joints, e.g. the tibial plateau distal to the anteromedial aspect of the knee joint line). The location should be chosen for its segmental effects, as indicated in Table 19.3. Then advance the needle tip until it touches the periosteum and just tap the periosteum a few times before removing the needle. It is important to take care not to use more than a few touches, since periosteal pecking can produce strong reactions, especially in younger patients. We advise practitioners to gain skill in handling needles in different tissues before they attempt periosteal pecking.

Another strong form of stimulation is deep painful needling used to activate descending inhibition. Common points are ST37 (for shoulder pain) and LR3 (for headache). The technique is an exaggeration of normal manipulation of a deep needle; the needle must be in muscle and is twisted to and fro as energetically as the patient can tolerate – having of course been forewarned.

Electroacupuncture

ORIGINS

EA developed in its modern form in China in the 1950s, specifically for use in surgical operations. When acupuncture was first used for analgesia, the anaesthetists had to continue to rotate needles manually throughout the operation, so they developed EA apparatus to relieve themselves of this chore. Although EA analgesia was initially used quite widely in China and caused a great deal of interest in the West, subsequently a clearer picture of its true value has emerged. EA analgesia may help reduce the requirement for intraoperative and postoperative analgesic drugs, but does not on its own produce a response reliably. Some patients gain a considerable rise in pain threshold, others none at all.

The decision to use EA in practice is personal. Some practitioners argue that EA goes against the spirit of a 'natural' therapy and that they can achieve all the results they need with manual needling alone. Other acupuncturists find EA useful, particularly for patients with chronic nociceptive pain who have failed to respond to one or two sessions with manual needling and for central stimulation (Fig. 15.3). Other possible roles for EA are as an adjunct to surgical analgesia and in treatment of drug addiction.

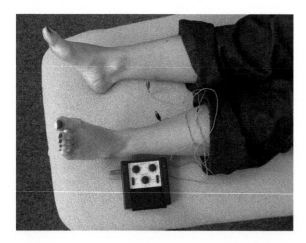

Figure 15.3 Electroacupuncture being given via a pair of leads attached to SP6 on each leg.

MECHANISMS

Broadly speaking, different frequencies of EA release different opioid peptides. We owe much of our knowledge on this subject to Ji-Sheng Han, who noticed that acupuncturists vary the way they stimulate needles with spinning or thrusting manoeuvres, sometimes fast and sometimes slow. Han chose the frequencies of 2 Hz and 100 Hz to represent the extremes (Han, 2004). But now we tend to refer to low frequency as 1–15 Hz, which may be the equivalent of muscular exercise, and high-frequency stimulation as 80 Hz or upwards, similar to that used in TENS. Specifically to regulate the autonomic system, a combination of low and intermediate frequency outputs (e.g. 2–4 Hz, 10–15 Hz) is probably best.

Han and colleagues showed that 2 Hz stimulation induces analgesia by release of β-endorphin, enkephalin and orphanin and their effect on μ receptors, and that high-frequency stimulation releases dynorphin, which stimulates kappa receptors (see Table 5.1). EA of 10–15 Hz induces a limited release of both enkephalin and β-endorphin and may be an optimal range for autonomic modulation (Stener-Victorin et al., 2003). In a comprehensive review of their findings, Han suggests that the greatest short-term analgesic effect is achieved by combining 2 Hz and 100 Hz (Han, 2004). Clinical research in patients with pain has suggested that the effect of 2 Hz is longer lasting than that of 100 Hz (Thomas et al., 1995).

The clinical effects of acupuncture in terms of pain relief and autonomic modulation probably depend on activation of deep Aβ and Aδ/type III fibres from muscle (Andersson and Lundeberg, 1995).

APPLICATION AND SAFETY

EA should not be used if the patient is at all nervous about electrical stimulation. In the United States it is not permitted to connect needles across the head or neck. Do not use EA in areas of sensory denervation. Readers should consult a freely accessible paper (Cummings, 2011), which discusses the safe application of EA in detail.

When intending to use EA, plan the placement of needles so that pairs can be connected together by pairs of leads from the apparatus. When deciding the depth and angle of the needles, remember that they will have to support the weight of the lead. Also, take the effect of muscle contraction into account, which can vary in different locations of the body and with different positions.

This all requires more care and consideration of factors in the patient (e.g. presence of implantable cardioverter defibrillator, ICD) and factors in the location (e.g. laryngeal muscles or carotid sinus) and needs greater knowledge of anatomy than manual acupuncture (Cummings, 2011).

Most apparatus offers three or four pairs of leads that can be connected at the same time. It is not easy to give comprehensive advice on the practical aspects in a book, and courses on EA are available. For treating areas of pain, the needles can be connected across the site in order to 'flood' the area with current. When treating an MTrP, one lead attaches to the needle in the point, and its pair attaches to a neutral needle at any other site.

A wise practitioner double-checks that the apparatus is switched off before connecting the leads to the needles, then gradually increases the strength of treatment while checking what the patient feels. If a needle is close to a motor nerve, muscle contraction may start very suddenly with a small increase in current, in which case the needle should be repositioned. The two parameters that can be controlled are the frequency and the intensity:

- *Frequency.* This usually ranges from 2–80 or 100 Hz. The most common arrangement is 3-second periods alternating between 2–4 Hz and 80–100 Hz. This pattern is designed to prevent nerve accommodation and to maximize the variety of neurotransmitters released.

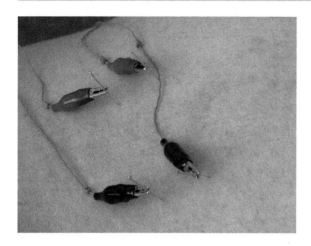

Figure 15.4   Electroacupuncture being used to treat facet joint pain.

Laboratory research suggests that intermediate frequencies (10–15 Hz) are optimal for autonomic modulation, so some practitioners choose to use 2–4 Hz with 10–15 Hz.

- *Intensity* of the electric current is usually between 0.5 and 20 mA, though usually the current is below 6 mA. Increase the intensity from zero slowly, firstly until the patient is aware of it and then further until it either causes muscle twitch or becomes as much as the patient can tolerate comfortably. When using two alternating frequencies, the patient may sense one frequency but not the other; this is where it is particularly useful if the apparatus allows separate intensity settings for each frequency.

Treatment is usually given for about 20–30 minutes. The response may tail off after the first few minutes, in which case the intensity must be increased again. Some patients may be willing and able to adjust the intensity for themselves. Occasionally, the intensity suddenly becomes strong – usually because the patient has moved, presumably bringing the needle closer to a nerve, so patients need to be informed about this possibility and told to reduce the intensity as rapidly as possible. Figure 15.4 shows EA being used to treat facet joint pain.

It is clear that EA applied across the thorax can affect the function of implantable medical devices such as ICD (Cummings, 2011). It may be acceptable to use EA in the limbs only, for example, but it is wise to consult the patient's cardiologist. It is also sensible not to give EA across the chest in the absence of devices, as there is a small but unknown risk of affecting the heart's conducting system. Calculations show that EA only generates an electrical charge around the heart of one-tenth the maximum recommended by the FDA. But the factors that control the intensity of the electrical field – type of current, skin thickness, needle type and depth of insertion – are still not known, so it is sensible to be cautious.

Do not connect needles electrically across the thorax (either on the chest wall or from arm to arm).

EA should also be used cautiously in patients with epilepsy, since sensory stimulation is very occasionally associated with a seizure. Needles should be placed where they do little damage in the case of a seizure, and patients with epilepsy undergoing EA should not be left alone.

EA to the scalp has been reported to cause angina pectoris. The symptoms recurred when the treatment was repeated, but no mechanism has been offered to explain this observation.

MOXIBUSTION

It is worth noting that thin myelinated nerve fibres also serve thermoreceptors that respond to warmth (not painful heat, which activates C fibres). The ancient therapy *moxibustion*, applying heat through burning a dried leaf (*moxa*) on the skin, is often considered as part of acupuncture. However, it could be risky to use moxa because it releases some toxic particulates. If heat is needed, infrared lamps can be used instead.

Individual patient sensitivity

Patients vary in their response to acupuncture, and some readily experience feelings of fatigue or malaise or a worsening of symptoms, as we discussed in the section on strong reactors in Chapter 14.

There is no definite way to anticipate who will react strongly, so the most sensible approach is a therapeutic trial with all patients; do not overstimulate on first treatment and then, if there has been no reaction, increase the strength of subsequent treatments. As a general guideline, it would usually be safe to start with no more than four or five needles, stimulated once, and not left longer than 10 minutes.

A few patients will have a severe reaction even to this cautious treatment, and then it is sensible to discuss with them the therapeutic options: either to give a lighter treatment next time (down to the bare minimum treatment with one small diameter needle retained for only 30 seconds) or to abandon treatment.

Managing the course of treatment

Acupuncture is often given as a course of treatment during which its effects accumulate. However, relatively acute musculoskeletal conditions, including MTrPs and other soft-tissue injuries that have failed to heal after (say) 6 weeks, may respond after just one or two treatments.

Second and subsequent treatments are guided by the response to earlier treatments. Most frequently, your patient will have noted some benefit, but it probably did not last. Repeat the treatment with a slightly increased dose to achieve cumulative benefit for more profound and longer-lasting effects.

For most conditions, patients and practitioners should be prepared to commit themselves to a course of about six to eight treatments – fewer if symptoms are of recent onset and limited to one area but more for chronic or extensive conditions. When pathology such as arthritis is present, treatment will probably have to be continued with 'top ups' at increasing intervals, initially monthly but then less frequently.

There is increasing interest in self-acupuncture for long-term conditions, among patients who are deemed capable and in conditions deemed suitable. Practitioners should gain some experience before considering teaching it to their patients.

Not all patients respond to acupuncture, of course. If there is no response to the first session, check the history and examination, then increase the strength of treatment. If there is still no response, it is worth modifying the treatment approach appropriately – adding extrasegmental or central points, for example, or adding EA. If there is no sign of response within the first four sessions, most practitioners will abandon acupuncture, though some argue that a few patients may not start to respond until they have had six sessions.

If you are treating a patient with cancer who suddenly stops responding to treatment that previously was effective, then consider the possibility that this is a sign of increasing tumour burden or recurrence.

Summary

This chapter describes the basic acupuncture technique and how to modify this technique to increase or decrease the dose of treatment, as required for each individual patient. The aim is to give sufficient dose to achieve a response, but not so strong that it produces a reaction. The dose can be tailored to the individual clinical circumstances in a number of ways, including the type and number of acupuncture point, needle type and number, depth of insertion, amount of stimulation, and the duration of treatment. Furthermore, the standard needling technique can be modified for inactivating myofascial trigger points, for superficial (minimal) needling and for periosteal pecking. Electroacupuncture (EA) is mainly used for central stimulation and to treat chronic pain and other conditions. Courses of treatment are typically three to eight sessions.

Safe needling

CONTENTS

Introduction

It is hardly necessary to emphasize the importance of safety, which should become integral to the practice of acupuncture. This chapter should be read in conjunction with the lists of overall contraindications and precautions in Chapter 14, Preparation for treatment. Advice is given on particular rules and techniques that are designed to avoid the most common adverse events that are reported in the literature.

TREAT PATIENTS WHO ARE LYING DOWN

The final preparation before needling patients is to position them correctly. Ideally, they should be lying down at least for the first treatment, to avoid fainting. Fainting can cause serious consequences (including seizure), and it also interrupts treatment and upsets patients. Occasionally, it may be impossible to gain access to the points that are needed, for example, the neck and shoulders, when the patient is supine. In these cases patients may be treated cautiously while they are sitting on the couch so that they can be laid flat immediately if they feel faint. Check the face for pallor or sweating and the pulse for bradycardia. If you need to lie the patient down, remove all needles instantly.

Treat patients while they are lying down, at least for the first treatment.

Equipment and administration

HANDLING NEEDLES

In most cases, needles are used once and then disposed of in the sharps bin. In the case of brief needling (e.g. treating MTrPs), then you may reinsert a needle, although beware that it rapidly

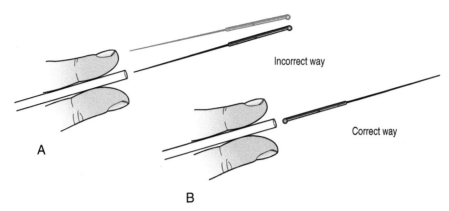

Figure 16.1 Diagram showing the risk of needle-stick injury on resheathing a needle; always resheathe the handle first.

becomes blunt and more painful when it crosses the skin and fascial layers. If a guide tube is used, the needle must be resheathed – handle first, not sharp end first, to avoid needle-stick injury (Fig. 16.1).

As a general principle, a needle should be in its original packet (unopened); in your hand in the guide tube, with the sharp end facing the patient; in a suitable point in the patient (during treatment); or in the sharps box. No needle should be left out of its packet lying unattended on any surface. Do not keep a patient's needles between treatment sessions, because the small savings in cost does not justify the risk of cross-infection associated with errors of handling. Guide tubes should not be shared between patients, again because of the small risk of cross-infection, so dispose of them after each patient contact.

FORGOTTEN PATIENTS

Another event that is embarrassingly common is forgetting a patient who is being treated in a side-room. It is easy to see how this can occur: a doctor, for example, in primary care is running a busy surgery and puts a patient in the side-room to allow more time for the acupuncture treatment. The doctor is called away on an urgent visit, and the patient is forgotten.

If the patient is treated in a side-room, install a system so that the patient can call for help. It is also wise to set up a reminder system in the main surgery to indicate that the side-room is occupied by a patient with needles.

Reducing the risk of trauma

Serious trauma is usually caused by inserting a needle either in the wrong place or in the right place but too deeply – both of which are avoidable. The following sections are organized according to the structure at risk. This chapter does not claim to be totally comprehensive; for example, it does not address all the risks associated with all acupuncture points, only those that are likely to be used by the beginner. It does assume some knowledge of anatomy and readers are also recommended to study carefully three articles that discuss details of human anatomy specifically for the acupuncturist (Peuker and Cummings, 2003a, 2003b, 2003c). Ultimately, the responsibility for safe practice rests with the practitioner.

BLOOD VESSELS

In the skin, reduce the risk of bleeding by avoiding needling into visible veins and by paying attention to swift, clean insertion and removal. Stop any bleeding quickly in the normal way by pressing with a clean swab or tissue and elevating the part, as appropriate. Haematomas can be uncomfortable and unsightly, especially in the neck and face. Have a swab ready to press any speck of blood after removing the needle. You should press on a bleeding spot for up to 2 minutes to reduce the likelihood of a bruise.

It is important to avoid needling larger blood vessels, particularly at the elbow and popliteal fossa. This is not just because of the risk of bleeding; in fact, serious bleeding is rare since the needle makes a clean hole, provided the limb has not moved too much while the needles were in position (e.g. electroacupuncture can make the part twitch), and bleeding is usually easily staunched by pressure. However, arterial damage from needles has occasionally been reported to cause traumatic aneurysms. Acupuncture to BL54/40 in the popliteal fossa caused an aneurysm of the popliteal artery that resulted in persistent symptoms of intermittent claudication. Similarly, a retroperitoneal haematoma has been reported as a result of bleeding from renal artery aneurysms that were produced by deep lumbar needling for back pain, and in another case the aorta was needled directly. Needless to say that all these incidents were avoidable.

Before needling near a superficial artery, always identify the position of the artery by feeling for the pulse.

Deep vein thrombosis has also been reported at the site where a patient had been treated with acupuncture. Clearly this is difficult to prevent, although the less mobile patients should be encouraged to move actively after treatment.

The vertebral artery is vulnerable to needling of GB20 (for point locations, see Chapter 19) and possibly BL10 in patients with slim necks, in whom the distance from the skin is less than the usual 4–6 cm; at GB20, a needle should not be inserted deeper than 3 cm in these patients and should be angled upwards towards the base of the occiput – and towards the contralateral eye.

HEART

The blood vessels on the surface of the heart are within the reach of a standard acupuncture needle. If these vessels are penetrated, they may bleed into the pericardial space where pressure rapidly builds up – a condition known as 'cardiac tamponade', which is likely to be fatal. There are reported cases and even a death from tamponade after acupuncture. Practitioners must be very clear that they know where their needles risk touching the heart:

- between the ribs over the anterior chest
- through sternal foramina (congenital abnormality)

Some 5–8% of the population have a congenital abnormality, the *foramen sternale*, which occurs when the two sides of the sternum fail to join together completely during ossification (see Plate 12). Usually this occurs at the fourth intercostal space, where the acupuncture point CV17 is located. When a foramen is present, the heart is only about 15–25 mm below the skin surface in slim patients, well within reach of the standard acupuncture needle (measurements from Elmar Peuker). The distance from the skin to the posterior surface of the sternum in one slim woman who died of cardiac tamponade was measured at postmortem and was between 13 and 19 mm. A foramen abnormality does not show on normal chest x-ray films, only on CT, and cannot reliably be detected by palpation. Therefore CV17 must always be needled either superficially or obliquely at a maximum angle of 30° to the sternum.

Although tamponade has been reported from a needle between the ribs, practitioners should not in any case be needling between the ribs on account of the much more common risk of pneumothorax.

PERIPHERAL NERVES

Very occasionally, needling produces local symptoms – usually numbness or motor weakness, occasionally pain – that may persist for several weeks, presumably from neuropraxia. It is not clear why this happens in some cases, and it seems unavoidable. It may be commonest at LI4.

One place where needle injury can affect nerve function is the common fibular nerve, close to GB34, where it can cause foot-drop. Sometimes the sciatic nerve is needled directly when treating the piriformis muscle, or GB30 or BL54, causing sharp shooting pain, though rarely any loss of function. The median nerve is easily reached by a deep needle at PC6. In all such cases, the needle should be withdrawn from the nerve immediately, and the patient reassured. It seems likely that acupuncture needles penetrate nerves fairly frequently but only rarely do any harm.

SPINAL CORD AND BRAINSTEM

The spinal cord and roots of the spinal nerves are vulnerable to deep needling at the paravertebral bladder and *Huatuojiaji* points, which should therefore be needled in a mediocaudal direction (e.g. towards the midline and towards the feet). In individuals of normal physique, the spinal cord is about 25–45 mm deep from the surface in the thoracic region and about 55 deep in the low lumbar spine where the cauda equina takes the place of the spinal cord. In the midline (GV points), a needle angled in a cranial direction can pass between the overlapping spinous processes, so needles should be directed caudally. Lesions to the spinal cord have occasionally been reported in Eastern literature. These injuries produce focal neurological signs or paraplegia.

Immediately below the occiput, the brainstem and the cerebellum are vulnerable to injury during needling. Even though there may be a tradition of deep needling in this area, we strongly advise not to needle deeply and to direct the needle upwards (cranially, towards the base of the occiput) when needling in the midline (GV points). At GB20, needle upwards and medially, towards the opposite eye.

PLEURAE

The pleurae overlie the lungs but offer minimal protection against needle penetration. Pneumothorax is the most common serious or potentially serious event reported in association with acupuncture. The chest wall is about 20–40 mm thick in healthy people, but compression of soft tissues is likely to occur during needling, so a depth of 10–15 mm should be regarded as the maximum in places where there is no rib or scapula to protect the pleura. Pneumothorax is a particular risk for patients with cachexia or a thin chest wall, which is likely in anyone seeking treatment with acupuncture for chronic respiratory disease. In these cases no needle should go further than immediately subcutaneously. But paradoxically, pneumothorax is also a risk in the obese as it is difficult to judge the thickness of tissues.

A pneumothorax can be produced by needling anywhere within the surface anatomy of the lung, but particularly in the supraclavicular fossa, between the ribs and medial to the upper scapula.

When needling over the ribs, the risk must be reduced in one of three ways (Fig. 16.2):
1. fix the skin (and trigger or acupuncture point) between the fingers, with the fingers placed in the intercostal space on either side of the rib, and needle directly over the rib;
2. use only superficial needling;
3. insert the needle obliquely, at a tangent to the ribcage.

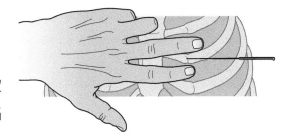

Figure 16.2 Diagram showing the technique for safe needling over the ribs; the trigger point has been fixed between the fingers, which are positioned over the intercostal spaces.

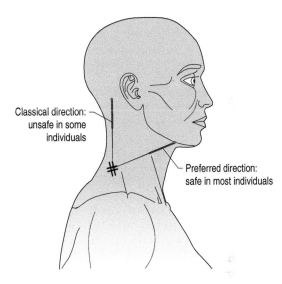

Classical direction: unsafe in some individuals

Preferred direction: safe in most individuals

Figure 16.3 Showing safe and dangerous approaches to needling GB21.

The point GB21 is frequently needled, and avoiding the pleura needs a particular technique, which is illustrated in Figure 16.3.

Another point to note in relation to pneumothorax is the difficulty making the diagnosis: pneumothorax may only present some time, up to 2 days, after the injury. Anyone with pain, cough or shortness of breath within 2 days of acupuncture should be suspected of having a pneumothorax. X-ray examination should be arranged urgently to make the diagnosis and guide the management. Tension pneumothorax has occasionally been described after acupuncture, and in this case, emergency hospital treatment will definitely be needed. Although we describe these serious cases, it seems possible that a number of minor cases of pneumothorax occur after acupuncture without being identified and resolve spontaneously.

ABDOMINAL ORGANS

Never needle right through the abdominal wall, or you are likely to cause peritonitis. It is rare to see a report of penetration of the abdominal organs, though a recent case was described of deep needling in the epigastric region causing an aortoduodenal fistula, which resulted in the patient's death. As a guide to the safe depth of needle insertion, the abdominal wall is approximately 20–40 mm thick in adults of normal weight. It becomes thinner when stretched and thinner still when compressed during needle insertion.

Reducing the risk of infection

There are two main possibilities of how patients could become infected through acupuncture: contamination by bacteria from the skin of the patient or the practitioner and transfer of blood-borne virus infection via needles contaminated with blood. Spreading infection between patients is eliminated by using single-use disposable needles.

HYGIENE AND SKIN PREPARATION

Practitioners should always clean their hands with soap and water or alcohol gel before treating a patient with acupuncture and between patients. This is reassuring to patients and reduces the very occasional risk that the hands may be contaminated with methicillin-resistant *Staphylococcus aureus* or hepatitis B virus from a previous patient. Alcohol gel is only an effective substitute for soap and water if the hands are not visibly soiled, as alcohol does not penetrate organic matter. Practitioners should cover any wounds or skin lesions they may have with waterproof dressing before treating patients.

Before inserting a needle, check that the patient's skin is clinically clean. There is no need to use alcohol swabs routinely before acupuncture, just as there is no need to use them before giving injections (Hoffman, 2001). Alcohol swabs do not reliably eliminate the bacteria on the skin surface and have little effect at all on the bacteria deep within the glands, follicles and crypts of the skin. Anyway, skin flora is generally of low pathogenicity. Alcohol can make needle insertion more painful. Long experience of injections without using swabs has shown no significant risk of infection. The number of bacteria that are likely to be inoculated on the tip of an acupuncture needle has been calculated to be well below that required to cause an infection in healthy patients (Hoffman, 2001). This probably explains why infection after acupuncture is much less common than might be expected.

However, occasional cases of infection have occurred, ranging from cellulitis to necrotizing fasciitis. Infection is more likely in certain sites and in debilitated or immunocompromised patients.

Long needles present a particular problem because the shaft needs to be supported while the needle is being advanced. Hold the shaft with a sterile swab or support it by using a shorter guide tube (a new one, not one used for another patient).

The consulting room should be kept in a high standard of cleanliness; for example, blood spillages should be cleaned promptly. All non-sharp contaminated items should be discarded in a clinical waste bag (usually a yellow bag).

VULNERABLE SITES AND VULNERABLE PATIENTS

Pay great attention in particular *sites* and in particular *patients*. The *sites* that are particularly vulnerable to infection include:
- cartilage of the ear (use a perpendicular insertion to avoid excessive damage to the cartilage);
- medial lower aspect of the leg, where varicose ulcers develop;
- a limb with (or prone to) lymphoedema after cancer – avoid needling this limb;
- a lower limb which has more than a trace of dependent oedema;
- any area where the blood supply is compromised, for example, by peripheral arterial disease;
- other sites where an infection would be particularly devastating, such as joint spaces (including joint effusions, when present), fracture sites and the meninges;
- where there is a foreign body such as a prosthetic joint.

The *patients* who are particularly at risk of infection include:

- immunocompromised patients, whether from conditions such as AIDS or as a result of immunosuppression therapy or cancer therapy, and
- those physically debilitated, for example, from chronic illness.

One report has suggested that a patient with diabetes mellitus was at an increased risk of infections from acupuncture, but this seems likely to be an isolated case. Apart from increased vigilance no special action is necessary in patients with diabetes.

However, serious infections have very occasionally been reported in previously healthy patients with no apparent risk factors: we have to put this down to misfortune. Most opportunistic infections with acupuncture are caused by the *Staphylococcus* group. However, *Clostridia* species have been cultured from abscesses in the cervical spine and the temporomandibular region, and *Mycobacteria* species are surprisingly common causes of skin infection.

BACTERIAL ENDOCARDITIS

Several cases of subacute bacterial endocarditis have been attributed to acupuncture. In some cases, the patients' heart valves were already abnormal following surgery or as a result of rheumatic fever. Some cases occurred after using indwelling needles, which are a recognized risk, but others occurred after sessions of normal body acupuncture, which is harder to explain. The full circumstances of the acupuncture are unknown in these cases, as they were reported by staff unconnected with the treatment. No particular precautions are currently advised with regard to sessions of body acupuncture treatment in patients with heart valve abnormalities.

Indwelling needles are contraindicated in patients with valvular heart disease (including prosthetic valve) or past history of endocarditis.

REDUCING BLOOD-BORNE INFECTION

In the past there were many cases in which hepatitis B virus was transmitted from one patient to another by acupuncture needles that were reused without being properly sterilized. One report highlighted the poor sterilization procedures used in some practices (Walsh, 2001). Epidemiological studies have shown a correlation between use of acupuncture and infection with hepatitis in some countries.

We are not aware of case reports of infection with hepatitis C attributed to acupuncture, though there is the possibility that patients have been infected but remain asymptomatic (Walsh, 2001).

Always use single-use disposable needles for acupuncture.

Similarly, there are four reports of the spread of HIV with acupuncture needles, though these cases are all 'probable' rather than 'certain' (White, 2004). Variant Creutzfeldt–Jakob disease is unlikely to be transmitted by acupuncture simply because the sites of infection (lymph nodes, tonsils, spleen and spinal cord) are not needled. However, the remote possibility of transmitting this disease, and the fact that the prion responsible is not killed by autoclaving, is another forceful argument against reusing needles.

Professional development

If something goes wrong, face up to it and discuss it frankly with the patient. Nobody gains if adverse events are concealed. Write a scientific report if it is serious or novel so that your colleagues can learn from it, and modify your practice procedures in light of the experience. Keep an eye on the literature for new reports of adverse events associated with acupuncture so that you can incorporate any recommended changes into your practice.

Summary

Safety should be integral to the practice of acupuncture. Patients should normally be treated supine. Single-use disposable needles are obligatory. Patients who are left relaxing in a side-room are at risk of being forgotten, and ways of avoiding this must be arranged.

Trauma to organs should be avoided; blood vessels, heart, peripheral and central nervous tissue, pleurae and abdominal organs are particularly at risk.

Practitioners must take great care to prevent avoidable cases of infection and wash their hands before treatment. The strictest aseptic technique is not necessary in normal cases. Particular care to avoid infection is recommended at the ear cartilage, in lymphoedema following surgery, gravitational oedema in the leg, anywhere the blood supply is compromised, and near prostheses. Patients who are immunocompromised or debilitated are also at risk. Patients with heart damage are at risk of endocarditis with indwelling needles. Practitioners should be aware of the risk of transferring blood-borne infection and take steps to avoid this.

Other acupuncture techniques

Introduction

Several different treatments have evolved under the heading of 'acupuncture and related techniques', including methods of continuous stimulation, different forms of stimulation, different models of treatment (microsystems) and electrical diagnostic methods.

The fact that a technique or piece of equipment is promoted and sold – or that it is included in this book – does not necessarily mean that it has been validated as an effective approach; most have not. Throughout the history of acupuncture, innovative practitioners have developed new ideas, probably for a variety of motives, including personal prestige and business reward. It is necessary frequently to remind ourselves that a novel and unusual technique in the hands of a committed practitioner can have powerful expectation effects; we do not support the promotion of any novel technique as an effective treatment until it has been properly evaluated.

One of our purposes in including these techniques in this introductory book is to give a brief overview with a neutral, or even slightly sceptical, attitude, so that beginners are cautioned not to spend large sums on apparatus that offers to cure every ill but then fails to live up to its promise.

However, there are two techniques that have some value: indwelling needles for continuous stimulation and auricular acupuncture as a particular form of nerve stimulation.

Continuous stimulation by indwelling needles

One traditional technique in acupuncture, especially when treating patients with chronic pain, is to increase the strength of stimulation by inserting indwelling needles, which continue to stimulate the point between the treatment sessions. Nowadays, the most common type of indwelling needle looks like the outline of a drawing pin (US 'thumbtack') as shown in Plate 9. These are also referred to as 'studs' especially when used in the ear. Various sizes are available, but the one with needle length of 2 mm is in most general use. Studs can be purchased with or without an adhesive dressing. Other methods are available for continuing the stimulation of the auricle, as we discuss below.

Of historical interest, the *umebari* technique from Japan was a rather notorious example of continuous stimulation: special, fine needles were inserted, then the handle portion was snipped off and the site massaged with the finger to drive the needle into the tissues. They were left there indefinitely. These *umebari* needles may be an incidental finding on x-ray examination many years later, or they can migrate around the body and cause trauma to distant tissues – kidneys and spinal cord have been reported. The Japanese professional acupuncture organizations effectively outlawed the procedure in 1976.

SAFETY OF INDWELLING NEEDLES

There are three principal concerns about the safety of indwelling needles:
1. They may cause local infection, particularly of the ear.
2. They may cause bacteraemia, which may lead to endocarditis in susceptible patients (see Chapter 13).
3. If they fall out, there is a risk of transmitting blood-borne infection through needle-stick injury. Many patients are unaware that they are carriers of hepatitis B or hepatitis C virus, and so any indwelling needle that they lose may constitute a significant risk to public health that is impossible to manage.

Because of these concerns, the UK professional body (British Medical Acupuncture Society) does not recommend the use of indwelling needles unless they are used in a way that you can be sure is safe. Firstly, check that the patient does not have valvular heart disease or any other increased risk from bacteraemia (e.g. from severe debilitation or compromised immunity); secondly, make sure either that you know the patient is not a carrier of hepatitis B or C virus, or that the needles will not fall out. In practice, then:
- ensure that the skin is clean before inserting the needle,
- cover the needle with a large and reliable dressing, for example, a clear surgical dressing (Plate 10),
- instruct the patient fully on the reasons to make sure the needle is not lost.

Full details and instruction sheets are provided in a review paper (Filshie et al., 2005). Devices, such as beads and seeds, that provide sustained acupressure rather than acupuncture are likely to be much safer (see Approaches to continuous stimulation), but may be less effective.

Auricular acupuncture

Auricular acupuncture forms a special subsection of acupuncture; its theory and practice as well as the necessary precautions are sufficiently different from body acupuncture to justify its own section here, but there is only room to touch on part of the whole subject.

BACKGROUND AND CONCEPTS

A French acupuncturist, Dr. Paul Nogier, discovered that local natural healers treated chronic back pain by cauterizing a particular area of the ear. Then, when one day the sun was shining

Phase I pattern | Phase II and III patterns | Phase IV pattern

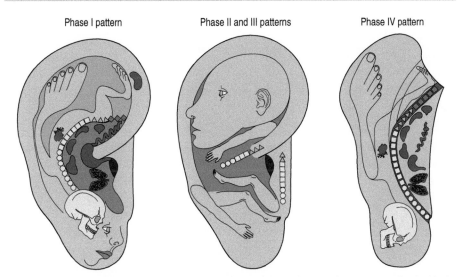

Figure 17.1 Different patterns of the supposed somatic representations on the ear, according to Nogier (*Reproduced with permission from Olson, T., 2003. Auriculotherapy Manual. Churchill Livingstone, p. 73.*)

across a patient's ear casting shadows, he noticed that the cartilage in that area consisted of a regular series of lumps that reminded him of the sacral spine. This gave him the idea that there might be some correlation between the ear and the rest of the body. He started examining the ears of all his patients, looking for a correlation between any spots, redness or tenderness in the ear and the patient's medical problem. He eventually derived the idea that the whole body is represented on the ear. This idea was soon adopted by the Chinese, acupuncturists throughout the world, and even the World Health Organization.

We are not convinced of the association and are reminded of the fairy tale story of the Emperor's new suit. He ordered his tailor to make the perfect suit, but they found it impossible. Rather than admit it, they presented him with a set of invisible clothes, telling him that it was made of special cloth which was invisible to anyone who was stupid. The Emperor, so conscious of his image as to be devoid of common sense, believed them. His advisors also said they were convinced by the tailors' descriptions of the beautiful patterns and the intricate weave, since they were driven by the fear of being labelled as stupid if they could not see the clothes. The Emperor wore the (non-existent) clothes in public, and everyone collaborated in the charade for fear of appearing stupid. It took the innocence of a small boy to announce: 'But he has nothing on at all'.

In charts of the original version, the body is represented upside down, like an inverted foetus; the head corresponds with the earlobe and the external auditory meatus with the umbilical cord. Nogier located the internal organs – the lung, heart, stomach, etc. – in the cavum concha, because it is usually innervated by the sensory branch of the vagus nerve. However, with further experience, Nogier found that this pattern did not always explain his findings in patients, so he produced alternative charts – either standing with the body represented erect or lying with the spine represented anteriorly – which could be used in patients whose ears did not match the first pattern; examples of these charts are shown in Figure 17.1, and readers can draw their own conclusions about the reliability of the method.

WESTERN MEDICAL AURICULAR ACUPUNCTURE

Even though the idea of the body being represented on the ear has no physiological basis and attempts to validate somatotopic representation have not been convincing, that is not to say that

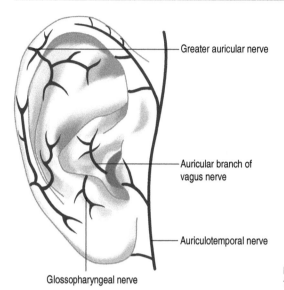

Greater auricular nerve

Auricular branch of
vagus nerve

Auriculotemporal nerve

Glossopharyngeal nerve

Figure 17.2 Diagram of the innervation of
the auricle.

acupuncture to the ear is of no value. Clinical experience suggests that stimulating the ear can produce useful clinical effects, even in cases that have not responded to standard, body acupuncture. The pinna is richly innervated by several nerves (shown in Fig. 17.2) and so is potentially a good site to stimulate the CNS in a direct, but rather general, way.

TREATMENT

There are several ways that practitioners of auricular acupuncture choose auricular points to needle: from the supposed correlations shown in published charts; or because they are tender; or because they show skin changes, particularly redness; or because they have a low electrical impedance. We cannot make firm recommendations about any of these.

Nogier used to insert the needle down to the cartilage and rotate it until the patient felt a burning sensation; this is not advisable because of the risk of injury to the cartilage and subsequent infection. Any stimulation with the needle should be gentle. Electrical stimulation can be used (though with caution in patients with epilepsy), but the current should not be connected from one side of the head to the other.

SAFE NEEDLING OF THE EAR

Particular safety precautions for auricular acupuncture include:
- Take particular care to avoid infection in the ear, as once present it can be difficult to treat and may produce deformation of the cartilage.
- Insert needles perpendicular and superficially to avoid damage to the cartilage.
- Do not use indwelling needles in any patient with valvular heart disease.

APPROACHES TO CONTINUOUS AURICULAR STIMULATION

Indwelling needles or studs placed in the external ear have been used either for treating chronic pain or for smoking cessation, as discussed below (p. 162). Indwelling needles are difficult to retain in the ear reliably, which means they carry a high potential risk of transmission of blood-borne

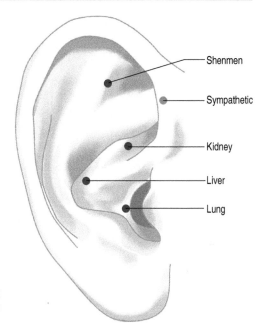

Figure 17.3 Points used in the NADA method of auricular acupuncture (Sympathetic point hidden in this view, on inner surface of helix).

viruses. Modern versions (see Plate 9 for an example) are acceptable, as they present the needle embedded in a plastic base to which the adhesive dressing is strongly attached.

It is important to regularly supervise patients wearing indwelling needles, as they carry a high risk of local infection because they maintain a track for bacteria to migrate beneath the skin, and because the ear cartilage has a poor blood supply.

Another type of needle was developed specifically for the ear, which has a barbed end to help retain it in the skin; this seems unnecessarily traumatic, so we do not include an illustration. This needle is also magnetic and is supposed to be stimulated by holding another magnet against it.

For these reasons, pressure devices are sometimes used, such as *Vaccaria* seeds (Plate 11) and special small stainless steel balls, held in place by adhesive tape. In our experience, even these are not entirely free of the risk of local infection. Also, very occasionally they become deeply embedded and covered in a flap of skin, making removal difficult. Another problem is that auricular acupressure seems less effective than acupuncture.

NADA TECHNIQUE

One particular technique of auricular acupuncture is currently in widespread use in the United States and Europe for treatment of opioid and cocaine dependence (Brumbaugh, 1993). It evolved after an anaesthetist in Hong Kong, Prof. Wen, used electroacupuncture (EA) at auricular points for surgical analgesia in patients who happened to be addicted to opioids; he noticed that they hardly experienced any withdrawal symptoms in the postoperative period (Wen & Cheung, 1973). Over time, the therapy spread to the United States and became what is known as the 'NADA' (National Acupuncture Detoxification Association) technique. EA across the head was not favoured in the United States, so a manual technique was used. Conventional acupuncture needles are placed in five points in both ears (Fig. 17.3), while the patient sits in a chair in a quiet relaxing environment for up to 45 minutes, generally in a group with other addicts. Treatment is offered on a drop-in basis, and recovered addicts are trained to apply the treatment, keeping staff costs low.

The place of this treatment has always been clearly elucidated by Michael Smith, who was responsible for introducing it (Brumbaugh, 1993). He believes that the main value of auricular acupuncture in detoxification is to attract addicts with a therapy that helps them relax. In this way, they gain trust in the healthcare providers and are more likely to enrol in the various services that offer help in facing the problems associated with their dependency. Smith insisted that the NADA therapy on its own is not likely to be sufficient in achieving abstinence, and his view has been supported by the majority of the evidence from clinical trials.

SMOKING CESSATION

Auricular acupuncture has also been widely adopted to help smokers quit smoking. The auricular points Lung and Shenmen (see Fig. 17.3) have been commonly used, and although evidence suggests that acupuncture at the correct site is no better than acupuncture at an incorrect site, acupuncture anywhere (in the ear) is clearly better than doing nothing to help the patient. The effect is not likely to be point-specific.

Some studies have used indwelling needles (studs) or acupressure devices, as described previously. The device is fitted on the quit-date, and the smokers are instructed to press the device with their finger whenever they feel cravings. Current evidence suggests this is the form of acupuncture most likely to help smokers quit. There is some evidence to suggest that this stimulus may affect the release of dopamine in the nucleus accumbens, but whether that is the true mechanism of action, or whether acupuncture is simply a distraction, it hardly matters if it helps achieve such an important target as stopping smoking.

Other stimulation techniques

ACUPRESSURE

Acupressure involves stimulating the body, usually at acupuncture points, with pressure from fingers, elbows or special devices. Various different approaches have originated in China, India, Korea and Japan, and they may have specific names, for example, 'Shiatsu'. Traditionally, hard wooden rods were used to apply real pressure! Some practitioners regard acupressure as a therapy in its own right, separate from acupuncture, though they often use traditional Chinese methods of diagnosis and treatment. The pressure used is quite considerable, and patients may feel bruised afterwards.

Sustained acupressure can be used for continuous stimulation, as a safer alternative to indwelling needles, discussed previously. The traditional method involved taping seeds of *Vaccaria* to auricular points (see Plate 11). Presumably these seeds were chosen because they were an appropriate size.

More recently, after it was demonstrated that PC6 acupressure can reduce nausea particularly in pregnancy, special elasticated wristbands with a pressure dome have been available (Fig. 17.4). They are also promoted for seasickness, and similar wristbands are sold that stimulate HT7 with the aim of treating insomnia, though there has been no validation of this claim.

MOXIBUSTION

Moxibustion is a traditional treatment used to warm either the needle or the skin itself (Plate 13). Moxa is a cotton-wool-like material made from the leaves of *Artemisia vulgaris*, which smoulders continuously rather than flaring up. It can be supplied:

- as loose 'punk', which is pressed round the needle handles or rolled into small *cones* burnt on the skin, either directly or on a slice of ginger;

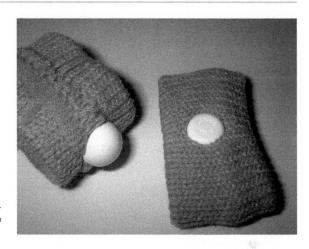

Figure 17.4 Photograph of commercially available wristband designed to apply pressure at PC6.

- rolled into a moxa *cigar*, the glowing end of which is held close to the acupuncture point, with or without the needle in situ.

We do not recommend the use of moxa. It constitutes a significant risk of burning the skin, it makes an all-pervading, unpleasant smell, and releases potentially harmful particulates. Traditionally in China, moxa was allowed to burn itself out on the skin, causing full-thickness blistering and permanent scar formation. Infrared lamps are used to warm the area around needles, as a kind of modern version of moxa. This method is very common in contemporary TCM practice.

PLUM-BLOSSOM NEEDLE

Plum-blossom needles consist of a number of short needles held close together with a long flexible plastic handle. This type of needle was used in the past as a local treatment to provide repeated stimulation to an area to produce erythema or bleeding. The original plum-blossom needle was impossible to sterilize adequately, but disposable versions are now available.

LASER 'ACUPUNCTURE'

Low-level lasers (i.e. lasers below the intensity that is needed to heat tissue) have been shown to have physiological effects, particularly in promoting the healing of skin ulcers. The light is directly absorbed by cells, but laser beams have not been shown to stimulate nerve endings. Acupuncturists became interested in lasers at the time of the initial AIDS scare in the 1980s, in the hope that they would offer an effective replacement for acupuncture needles. Another thing that made them popular at that time was significant reduction in their cost. Lightweight and cheap crystals that produced light of a single wavelength became available and soon replaced the original heavyweight laser generators.

Some early studies seemed to show that laser therapy could have systemic effects, and the idea developed that lasers could stimulate acupuncture points. Evidence shows that laser acupuncture can inhibit nerve conduction. There are theoretical doubts about this. The red laser, which was shown to have physiological effects, does not penetrate the skin more than a few millimetres, since it is absorbed by haemoglobin. The energy reaching the tissues may not be sufficient to adequately stimulate nerve endings. Infrared laser may penetrate further, but there is no clear evidence to show that this wavelength has beneficial physiological effects.

There is still debate between practitioners on the optimal dosage (wavelength, power and duration) of laser therapy that should be used at acupuncture points, but the evidence clearly shows that a dose of at least 0.5 J per point and power of 10 mW or more are necessary to obtain clinical effects. Double-blinded studies using these parameters have shown positive results. The final verdict on whether laser may be effective in conditions such as headache and neck pain is still unknown. We suggest that practitioners should wait for more definitive evidence and guidance before investing in laser as an alternative for needles.

TRANSCUTANEOUS ELECTRICAL NERVE STIMULATION

Transcutaneous electrical nerve stimulation (TENS) is sometimes included in descriptions of acupuncture. It consists of the application of electrical current to the body through carbonized rubber pads. The original frequency used was high, about 100 Hz or more, and only strong enough to produce a light tingling sensation. Later, the so-called 'acupuncture-like TENS' was developed using much lower frequencies (about 2 Hz) at strong enough intensity to cause muscle contraction.

In reality, even 'acupuncture-like TENS' is different from acupuncture as presented in this book. TENS was developed from theoretical considerations (i.e. knowledge that stimulation of Aβ fibres could inhibit pain transmission); acupuncture was developed by clinical tradition. TENS is used to treat pain, whereas acupuncture treats other symptoms too. TENS has an immediate effect, which is short term and has to be repeated or used continuously, but acupuncture appears to have more lasting effects.

GOLD AND SILVER NEEDLES

Some manufacturers still provide needles made of gold or silver, which were supposed to 'stimulate' and 'drain' the patient's energy respectively. However, this interpretation is probably the result of a mistranslation from Chinese. Needles made of gold or silver are now virtually redundant since they require autoclaving and rapidly become blunt and painful to insert.

Other acupuncture microsystems

Apart from auricular acupuncture, several other systems that have been promoted use the concept of somatotopic representation, that is, the body represented somewhere in miniature form, the homunculus. Inserting needles into the appropriate site is supposed to have an effect on the remote part, and in some cases the system is also used for diagnosis. The basis of these microsystems is actually a distortion of Sherington's original concept of the homunculus in the brain. He demonstrated that the body is represented on part of the cerebral cortex through somatotopically distributed neural connections.

NEW SCALP ACUPUNCTURE OF YAMAMOTO

In Japan, Yamamoto developed a homunculus situated over the temple. This was a serendipitous finding: he was using acupuncture for treating various deficits in poststroke patients, found he was wasting time waiting for patients to undress for body acupuncture, and hit on the idea of asking them just to remove their hats. In a busy clinic, this simple manoeuvre saves a good deal of time. Scalp acupuncture was already used for patients with stroke in some parts of China, usually involving threading a long needle subcutaneously over the affected area. Yamomoto evolved the idea that different points on the scalp represent different organs, reminiscent of Nogier's auricular charts. He extended the application of NSAY (new scalp acupuncture of Yamamoto) to other medical conditions, yet the therapy remains largely unevaluated.

KOREAN HAND ACUPUNCTURE

Korean hand acupuncture developed in 1971 and uses a slightly different idea: in this case, every meridian is supposed to be represented on the hands, including the conventionally named points. Treatment of the hands alone is supposed to be sufficient.

INTERPRETATION

In summary, it seems possible that microsystems could be interpreted simply as an expression of the fact that needle treatment (almost) anywhere can produce valuable central effects, some specific and some non-specific. These effects rely on stimulating nerve endings, and the ear and hand are richly innervated. We have reservations about the microsystem concepts described here and do not believe that the claims of somatotopic representation (i.e. body represented on one limited area) have been subjected to sufficient scrutiny in controlled trials.

Electrodiagnostic techniques

These techniques are quite distinct from EA treatment as described previously, which does not make any claims to diagnose patients.

ELECTROACUPUNCTURE AFTER VOLL

Voll was an electrical engineer who later studied biology and came across the concept of acupuncture points. While investigating their electrical properties, he developed an apparatus that could detect changes in skin resistance with pressure from a probe. The apparatus essentially consists of a Wheatstone bridge, but extra functions and sensitivities are claimed for it. In apparatus purchased on the open market, the circuitry is sealed with rubber to prevent examination. The EAV apparatus has stimulated many copies and 'developments', which add extra features and make additional claims. The makers of the apparatus claim it can measure the electrical performance of acupuncture points, which can be used to detect the underlying condition of individual organs of the body. A far as we are aware, the only rigorous investigation of this apparatus that has been carried out (testing how reliably it could detect allergies) was clearly negative (Lewith et al., 2001).

RYODORAKU

In Japan in about 1950, Yosio Nakatani claimed to find a line of increased electroconductivity in the skin in meridians that related to diseased organs. Measurement of all the points, generally the terminal points on fingers and toes, is said to provide a diagnosis of the autonomic disturbance underlying the condition. Electrical stimulation at those points is given with the aim of correcting the disturbance.

Summary

It is wise to adopt a cautious approach toward novel treatments until they have been properly evaluated.

Continuous stimulation with indwelling needles may enhance the effectiveness of acupuncture in chronic pain, and indwelling studs can be used. Indwelling needles should be used with caution as they carry significant risks of infection, including local sepsis, bacteraemia and blood-borne spread of infection to another person if they fall out.

Auricular acupuncture developed in France, and the original principle was that the body is represented (upside down) on the auricle. There is no known mechanism for this idea; however, the auricle is well innervated and likely to be a good site for stimulating the central nervous system. The NADA technique is widely used for treatment of drug dependence. Continuous stimulation with studs has been used for smoking cessation. Other stimulation techniques allied to acupuncture include acupressure, for example, wristbands for treating nausea; moxibustion, which has limited use in a modern clinic; laser 'acupuncture'; and transcutaneous electrical nerve stimulation (TENS). As these therapies do not involve needling, they have only a peripheral connection to acupuncture.

Further reading

Baxter, G.D., McDonough, S.M., 2016. Laser acupuncture. In: Filshie, J., White, A., Cummings, M. (Eds.), Medical Acupuncture: A Western Scientific Approach, second ed. Churchill Livingstone, Edinburgh, pp. 269–277.

A realistic description of the suggested physiology of laser acupuncture therapy, with evidence-based discussion of dosage, and the application of laser acupuncture in various indications together with the available evidence.

Johnson, M.I., Thompson, J.W., 2016. Transcutaneous electrical nerve stimulation (TENS). In: Filshie, J., White, A., Cummings, M. (Eds.), Medical Acupuncture: A Western Scientific Approach, second ed. Churchill Livingstone, Edinburgh, pp. 234–268.

A detailed exposition of TENS, covering historical background, principles, treatment plans and optimal technique, as well as research on clinical effectiveness and on mechanisms.

Usichenko, T., Anders, E.E., 2016. Auricular acupuncture. In: Filshie, J., White, A., Cummings, M. (Eds.), Medical Acupuncture: A Western Scientific Approach, second ed. Churchill Livingstone, Edinburgh, pp. 144–166.

A practical and evidence-based presentation of auricular acupuncture which covers its history and mechanisms, and uses for many conditions including anxiety and pain, particularly relating to surgery, as well as drug dependency and insomnia.

Treatment Manual

Treatment guidelines

Introduction

This chapter should not be applied on its own; it is intended to be used only in the context of the particular approach to acupuncture that has been described in this book. Do not look here for formulae for treatment. There is no such thing as 'standardized' treatment, formula, or prescription in acupuncture, any more than there is a standardized way to treat a respiratory infection – it all depends on the particular patient and their particular condition. You have discovered the principles of acupuncture in the previous chapters; here you will find some guidelines to point you in the right direction. Chapter 19 provides reference material to put these guidelines into practice. But it is still up to the acupuncturist to consider the actual patient and their individual case and then to apply common sense and clinical judgement in order to plan the best possible treatment. That is the art of medicine and also of acupuncture.

This chapter gives some guidelines on how to apply the principles to some common conditions. It is based, as always, on choosing the appropriate mechanism for the case. However, sometimes the cause of the clinical problem may not be clear-cut, and you may deliberately plan to combine several mechanisms. For example, you might choose a point because it has a local effect on the tissues as well as a segmental analgesic effect, or you might use a major point that covers both descending analgesia and central regulatory effects.

Our guidelines are mostly about pain, and particularly musculoskeletal pain. This is both because pain is the condition that acupuncture is most commonly used for and because in our experience it has the most predictable response and the best understood mechanisms.

Although our approach to acupuncture is based on the current understanding of its mechanisms, there is still room for intuition. For example, you may decide to place a needle in a muscle tissue that is found to be tender, even though it might not be easy to link the location directly with the clinical picture. A therapeutic trial is justified as long as the patient is closely observed and the trial abandoned if there is no response within a reasonable time. This is not an excuse to think that acupuncture is just some kind of art form that relies entirely on intuition – the fundamental approach to the patient should always be based on a reasoned argument.

Finally, if you make a clinical observation that is novel or does not seem to fit into the current understanding, you are strongly encouraged to report it in the acupuncture literature as a case history. The rich tapestry of individual histories is fertile and challenging ground for helping to develop and extend our understanding of this ancient therapy.

Summary of general treatment principles

SELECTING THE POINT

By the time you have conducted the history and examination you will probably have formed a conclusion about the cause of the problem, and which of the approaches the patient needs. Table 18.1 gives examples of the types of conditions in which the different mechanisms apply and the sort of locations where you may think about choosing points to needle.

Choose points that fit into more than one category if possible and, of course, you are not restricted to needling only classical points. However, only choose points that are in healthy tissue and have an intact nerve supply.

STIMULATING THE POINT

Stimulation is applied according to the type of mechanism that is to be activated, the nature of the patient and the patient's response. These are briefly summarized in Table 18.2.

TABLE 18.1 ■ Examples of conditions and point locations for different treatment approaches

Approach	Example of condition	Point location
Local	Local skin or other soft tissue condition	Within about 25 mm of the problem and about 20–50 mm apart
Myofascial trigger point (MTrP)	MTrP pain	Precisely on MTrP
Segmental analgesia inc. long-loop analgesia	Joint pain, other nociceptive pain	In same segment, or adjacent segments; paravertebral points for spinal conditions
Segmental autonomic effects	Bladder or bowel functional disorder	Abdominal points for abdominal visceral conditions
Descending analgesia (remote effect)	Shoulder pain	Special points (e.g. ST37 for shoulder pain)
Central regulatory	Pain with large affective component; conditions without pain	Major points, bilaterally

TABLE 18.2 ■ **Summary of methods of stimulation used in different treatment approaches**

Approach	Stimulation
Local analgesia	Needle subcutaneously and stimulate lightly
Myofascial trigger point	Needle accurately to obtain local twitch responses, repeat if necessary, fanning out needle direction, or needle superficially; electroacupuncture may be useful for chronic MTrPs
Segmental	Stimulate manually to elicit *de qi,* and maybe repeat stimulation at about 5 minute intervals, or use electroacupuncture for 10–20 minutes, or periosteal pecking
Descending analgesia (remote effect)	Stimulate manually strongly to elicit *de qi;* use electroacupuncture for 10–30 minutes
Central regulatory	Gentle manual stimulation to elicit *de qi,* or sometimes electroacupuncture; 20–40 minutes leaving the patient to relax

INCREASING THE DOSE OF TREATMENT

Start with slight underdosing, if anything, then increase the dose by:

- adding more points,
- manipulating the needles for longer and more than once,
- possibly retaining the needles for longer (though from clinical observation the duration seems to make little difference),
- adding electroacupuncture (EA),
- adding another treatment approach, such as periosteal pecking or auricular acupuncture.

Guidelines: musculoskeletal conditions

All guidelines are given with the usual caveat throughout this book. A standard medical diagnosis should be made in all patients before choosing acupuncture; acupuncture may relieve the symptoms of serious underlying disease temporarily and, thus, lead to delay in patients having the definitive treatment they need.

MYOFASCIAL TRIGGER POINT PAIN

When the history suggests myofascial trigger point (MTrP) pain – unilateral pain that fluctuates, often for no obvious reason – identify the area of pain and compare it with the charts in the next chapter. Search across muscle fibres with your finger to find the MTrP, as described in detail in Chapter 6, and needle as is described in Chapter 15. Also, try to identify which activities provoke the pain and advise the patient to modify the way they do them, or if necessary avoid them completely.

OSTEOARTHRITIS (OA)

- Start with a segmental approach using two to four local points, including at least one traditional point and perhaps a tender point near the joint line.
- Increase the dose by using more local segmental points and descending analgesia points – ideally, choose traditional points that are tender and are situated in the area of referred pain.

- If you find active MTrPs in the muscles that act on the joint, treat them.
- Periosteal pecking can be used in patients who appear less sensitive to needling or do not easily feel *de qi*, for example, on the greater trochanter for OA hip.
- Do not insert needles into the joint space.
- Do not expect complete relief in patients with serious joint destruction; there are finite limits to the potential of acupuncture, and it is no substitute for joint replacement surgery in advanced cases.

There follow some suggestions of traditional points that can be used to treat individual joints (see Chapter 19 for point locations):

- *Wrist* LU7
- *Base of thumb* LI4, TE5
- *Shoulder* LI15, SI11
- *Hip* GB30, GB29; distant segmental GB34
- *Knee* four local points, including ST36, ST33, SP10, SP9; distant descending analgesia LR3
- *Ankle* SP6, BL60, KI3, LR3.

SPINAL OR PARASPINAL PAIN (NECK, THORAX, LOW BACK)

Try to localize the main level of origin of the pain by history and palpation and to identify whether it is in the region of the spine or in the paravertebral tissues.

Examine for MTrPs that refer pain to the area, particularly in unilateral pain: they will most commonly be in trapezius for neck pain; rhomboids for thoracic pain; and erector spinae, quadratus lumborum or gluteus medius for pain in the lumbar region.

For spinal pain that is not due to MTrPs, use segmental points around the area of pain; mainly GV, *Huatuojiaji* and BL points, together with GB points in the neck and shoulders.

Reinforce or increase the effect by adding distant segmental or descending analgesia points, for example BL60.

Muscle spasm in patients with back pain can often be relieved swiftly by needling directly over or into the muscles involved, but this is likely to give only temporary relief if there is an underlying condition such as a prolapsed disc.

SOFT-TISSUE CONDITIONS

Lateral epicondylitis

Consider this first as a symptom of MTrPs in the extensor muscles, and supinator, and treat these in the usual way. If no MTrP can be found, or to increase the dose of treatment, use LI11, LI10 and add LI4 or periosteal pecking.

Medial epicondylitis

Similarly, search for MTrPs, but this time near the origin of the flexor group of muscles and pronator teres.

Shoulder pain

If pain is due to MTrPs arising from some episode when the muscles were overloaded, then acupuncture has a good chance of treating the pain successfully. However, classical 'frozen shoulder' is difficult to treat: the painful phase may be reduced in length, but it is not clear whether or not the time course of the restriction to the range of movement is reduced as well. EA is commonly used for chronic shoulder pain, and typical pairs of points would be LI15-LI16 and TE14-SI11.

Tenosynovitis, for example, de Quervain's

Treat local tender points and acupuncture points, but do not needle the ligament sheath – avoid direct needling of any acutely inflamed tissue.

Plantar fasciitis

This condition can be difficult to treat with acupuncture, but occasionally the pain in the foot is due to an MTrP in the medial head of gastrocnemius. If so, you should be able to reproduce the patient's pain complaint by pressing over the TrP. For true plantar fasciitis, try local classical points; the plantar fascia itself is painful to needle, and the skin of the heel pad is thick and tough. However, it may be possible to needle directly into the tender point using a medial approach.

Ligaments and tendons

Soft-tissue injuries that are slow to recover can be encouraged to heal by brief needling, often at the most tender point. Acupuncture is likely to produce analgesia lasting some hours, so the patient should be warned not to overstretch the tissue (e.g. by playing sports) and thereby risk further injury.

Non-cardiac chest pain

If non-cardiac chest pain is not due to gastrointestinal disease, fibromyalgia, or local conditions of the ribs, it is quite likely to be caused by MTrPs. Search for these in the pectoral muscles, mainly the pectoralis major, anywhere from the muscle attachment to the rib to the musculo-tendinous junction in the anterior axillary wall. Always consider the underlying lung – needle into tissue held in a pincer grip, directing the needle towards one of your own fingertips placed on the other side of a trigger point band, or onto a rib, or superficially (just into the first muscle layer).

Guidelines: other painful conditions

TENSION-TYPE HEADACHE

Examine the neck and shoulders for relevant MTrPs. They are likely to be found in the trapezii: these, and the posterior neck muscles and the suboccipital muscles, should be examined systematically. In addition, the sternomastoids refer pain to the temporal and ear regions. Sometimes the history of the localization of the pain will enable you to diagnose which particular muscle harbours the MTrP, from the diagrams in the next chapter. Examine the neck in the sitting position but treat the patient lying down; note that the MTrPs in postural muscles may not be so easy to find when lying down.

> Commonly used traditional points for tension type headache are GB20 and GB21.

LI4 and LR3 are useful descending analgesia points for tension-type headache and may have central regulatory effects that could be beneficial if anxiety is prominent. LI4 may sometimes be considered segmental as it stimulates the myotome T1, and the sympathetic (efferent) supply to the head comes mostly from the T1 segment.

MIGRAINE

The treatment of migraine involves finding and treating any relevant MTrPs in the neck and shoulders and GB20, GB21, as for tension-type headache, together with more emphasis on some major points for their central regulatory effect. Commonly used classical points are LR3 in particular and LI4. LR3 is used for traditional meridian reasons (LR and GB meridians are a *yin yang* pair); however, it probably works acutely on migraine via heterotopic noxious conditioning stimulation (HNCS) by creating a strong stimulus at the opposite end of the spinal inputs from the head.

ATYPICAL FACIAL PAIN

This may be due to undiagnosed MTrPs, so examine the masticatory muscles and the muscles of facial expression carefully; also consider primary MTrPs in upper trapezius. You may need to consult other texts for more detail on the pain referral patterns of individual muscles.

If no MTrPs can be found, then treatment should be directed to classical acupuncture points in the face together with GB20. GB20 is a point considered to be segmental for the whole of the head and face since it stimulates the myotome of C1, and the spinal trigeminal nucleus extends beyond C1 in the cord (perhaps as far as C4, though certainly to C2).

FIBROMYALGIA

Some patients clearly respond to acupuncture treatment so it is worth a trial. Temporary aggravations by acupuncture seem to be more common among patients with fibromyalgia than with other conditions, particularly from needling tender points in muscle – this is one condition where practitioners should be cautious of treating tender points (another is complex regional pain syndrome).

The wisest approach is to use gentle treatment initially on some major points in hands and feet, and, if possible, some points near the symptoms, but only if they are not too tender. Some authorities recommend only 30 seconds treatment with each needle. If this is enough to start a response, then this can be reinforced by gradually leaving the needles in place for longer. However, if there is no strong reaction to the first treatment, it is probably best to use EA – the present evidence suggests that this will be most beneficial.

Patients with fibromyalgia often have one or two distinct areas of myofascial pain, as well as the generalized soft-tissue pain. It is thought that targeting this myofascial pain may not only improve the localized pain, but may result in some general improvement in the condition. Treatment should be cautious initially since compliance will be reduced if postneedling soreness is excessive. It is also important to consider treating any visceral comorbidities, since improvement in these will reduce symptoms associated with fibromyalgia.

INTERMITTENT CLAUDICATION

Use the traditional points BL57 and major points on the feet, as well as any TrPs in the gastrocnemius and soleus muscles, and segmental points at L2 level. Any improvement in the condition is likely to be through reducing secondary myofascial pain rather than improved circulation.

Be aware that this condition tends to improve spontaneously somewhat in the period after first diagnosis, so do not be overeager in claiming to have cured the patient!

PHANTOM LIMB PAIN

Check for trigger points on the stump and treat them cautiously because of the risk of painful reaction. For neuroma pain, very gentle direct needling of the neuroma may be a useful technique to try after the more standard approaches suggested here. The most common approach is to use classical points in the residual limb or limb girdle and paravertebral points on the same side, or bilaterally.

Treat mirror points on the other limb – mirror images of the points in the area of pain – and consider auricular acupuncture.

TRIGEMINAL OR POSTHERPETIC NEURALGIA

Treat the segment above (or below) the affected segment or the segment on the opposite side (mirror points), for fear of a painful reaction to needling the affected segment. You may need to add EA.

If there is no response, then treat within the segment, but only gently at first.

COMPLEX REGIONAL PAIN SYNDROME AND RAYNAUD'S SYNDROME

Though the pathology of these two conditions is clearly different, they can be approached in a similar way, and a few patients with each condition will respond.

Choose local major points in the affected limb and limb girdle, but do not give strong treatment to sensitive sites, for fear of aggravating the symptoms.

Add paraspinal segmental needling to the relevant segments (see Fig. 16.14) to influence both the somatic segments and the segments responsible for the relevant sympathetic outflow.

Guidelines: abdominal symptoms

GASTROINTESTINAL SYMPTOMS

Acupuncture will mainly be symptomatic, directed to the relief of pain and dysfunction in conditions such as irritable bowel syndrome. The simplest and most effective approach is to needle tender points in the abdominal wall muscles (segmental approach) or strong abdominal points, such as CV12 and ST25. Major points in the lower limb, such as ST36, LR3, will have descending inhibitory and central regulatory effects.

BLADDER SYMPTOMS

As with gastrointestinal symptoms, needle the tender points over the lower abdominal wall for any bladder symptoms, such as irritative bladder. Add points over the sacrum (BL points) and several lumbar paravertebral points for the autonomic outflow, and pick up the sacral segments in the lower limb, for example, SP6, KI3, ST36, LR3. See also Tables 16.1 and 16.2.

Guidelines: conditions without pain

NAUSEA

Nausea due to pregnancy, surgery or chemotherapy can often be diminished by treatment with acupuncture, typically at PC6 and possibly ST36, although needle location may not be critical. Ideally, start the treatment before the onset of nausea. Unlike when treating pain, the relief of nausea does not seem to last more than a day or so; patients should either be treated quite frequently – say three times a week – or be shown how to use acupressure bands, which they should press to massage the wrist every 2 hours. CV12 is also used for nausea, but this point seems most relevant if there is some form of gastric irritation responsible.

HAY FEVER, ALLERGIC RHINITIS

Typical points used are LI20 and *Yintang, Taiyang* together with LI11 and ST36. Add LI4 and LR3 if needed to increase the dose.

Acupuncture may give instant relief for hay fever, presumably due to a local or regional sympathetic response on the blood vessels in the linings of the nose, and if repeated weekly about three times before the season it may prevent attacks altogether.

MENOPAUSAL HOT FLUSHES

Any general stimulation is likely to produce an effect in suitably responsive patients, typically LI4, SP6 and LR3. EA may have some benefit over manual needling.

BREATHLESSNESS

Breathlessness or dyspnoea can be associated with a number of serious medical conditions, and we are not suggesting acupuncture should be tried unless conventional treatment has been exhausted or is lacking. The circumstances in which this symptom is generally treated is part of palliative care of the patient with cancer affecting the lung or disabling chronic obstructive pulmonary disease. Points used are ASAD (two periosteal points over the manubrium); thoracic paraspinal points from T2 to T5; trigger points in shoulder girdle muscles, especially trapezius; and general points such as LI4.

TINNITUS

Tinnitus may rarely be a symptom of an MTrP in the deep portion of the masseter muscle or the clavicular head of sternocleidomastoid – likely clues are that the symptoms will fluctuate, are likely to be unilateral and are not associated with hearing loss. Persistent, continuous tinnitus has occasionally appeared to respond to local needling at SI19, GB20, etc., but RCTs have not shown specific effects.

ITCH

Sometimes pruritus responds to acupuncture – local needles surrounding any particular lesion and the usual major points for an overall effect. Be aware that generalized pruritis may be a sign of serious underlying pathology.

Safety first

We shall not repeat the advice on safe practice from other chapters of this book, but simply remind readers that they must constantly think of the patient's safety as well as the effectiveness of the acupuncture treatment.

Recording treatment

Records of treatment need to be as precise as possible, within the limits of the space available in clinical notes, indicating the points used, the amount of stimulation and the duration of needle retention. It is important to know what you have done at one treatment, so you can adjust it next time according to the response – which should also be recorded especially after the initial treatment.

Some standard symbols can be used as a kind of shorthand, as shown in Table 18.3. The points used can be written (or a small diagram if not a known point) with two circles above for bilateral treatment, and a single circle with the letter R or L after it for unilateral treatment; depth can be recorded as S for superficial, D for deep, and P for periosteal needling; some kind of scale such as x0 to x3 to indicate the amount of manual stimulation; EA for electroacupuncture; and the duration of needle retention, in minutes.

TABLE 18.3 ▪ **Examples of records of acupuncture treatment**

Treatment details	Shorthand record in notes
One needle inserted superficially at LI11 without stimulation, retained for 5 minutes	LI11 S1 x0–5'
Treatment of these four major points with deep needles given one stimulation and retained for 20 minutes	LI4, LR3 D4 x1–20'
Moderately strong manual needling at three points, retained for 20 minutes	ST36, SP9, SP10 D3 x2–20'
Strong periosteal needling to one point for 10 seconds (describe the point, e.g. tip of acromion, or draw small diagram)	P1 x3 –10''
Electroacupuncture given at stated frequencies for 30 minutes (drawing indicates location)	EA 2/15 Hz–30'

Reference charts: points and innervation

How to locate acupuncture points

MYOFASCIAL TRIGGER POINT PAIN REFERRAL PATTERNS

Ask the patients to delineate the area of their pain as precisely as possible, then look for the pattern on the appropriate chart. Myofascial trigger point (MTrP) diagrams include the site of the MTrP indicated with a cross-hatch symbol. The long strokes of the symbol indicate the muscle fibre orientation. The two-tone shaded areas are examples of possible pain referral patterns from the relevant TrPs. The darker areas indicate the more frequent sites of pain. Prepare your acupuncture needle so you can immediately treat any point(s) you find.

Feel the fibres under the fingertips, feeling for the taut band then for the most tender part of the taut band. Most muscles can be examined by flat palpation. Use pincer palpation for the anterior border of trapezius in the shoulder in slim individuals, the lateral fibres of the pectoralis major in the anterior axillary wall, and the sternocleidomastoid (gently).

TRADITIONAL ACUPUNCTURE POINTS

We have chosen a sample of points for this introductory book because they are either:
- major points for descending analgesia or central regulatory effects: LI4, TE5, PC6, LI11, ST36, SP6, KI3, BL60, LR3;
- useful in treating common conditions (round arthritic joints);
- illustrative of principles of locating points elsewhere (alongside the spine);
- at or close to common myofascial trigger points (e.g. GB21).

Readers who want to learn more traditional points (instead of using their fingers to find appropriate places to treat) can look in the texts listed at the end of this chapter.

BONY LANDMARKS

Classical points tend to be either dips into which the finger sinks naturally (ST36) or summits of a prominence, for example a bulging muscle (LI4). They often are described in relation to a particular skin crease or to a bony landmark – the prominence of the spinous processes, a joint line, the highest point of the femoral tuberosity. For those unfamiliar with superficial anatomy, we add some aide-memoire for identifying individual locations, where appropriate.

Find the actual point for inserting the needle by exploring with your finger for the most tender site. Myofascial trigger points need to be located by the special technique described in Chapter 6.

BODY MEASUREMENTS

The Chinese system of proportional measurement is still useful for finding some of the points. The Chinese argued that patients do not come in fixed sizes, so they divided each part of the body into a constant number of units. They called the unit *'cun'* (pronounced tsun), which is sometimes referred to as the 'Chinese inch'. For example, the middle phalanx of the middle finger is 1 *cun,* and the elbow crease to the wrist crease is 12 *cun* (Fig. 19.1). Points are best found by subdividing up the whole distance, but an alternative is to count *cun* from one end.

Conveniently, the fingers can be used in various combinations to make measurements (Fig. 19.2). For example, one important point, PC6 is located 2 *cun* up from the wrist. Although obviously it should be the patient's own hand that is used, in practice it is the examiner's hand that is often used after a quick comparison with that of the patient – which is fine because points really do not have to be located all that precisely.

Most points are found by measuring from a bony landmark using the fingers, but the abdomen is usually measured, at least in the axial direction, by using the fixed divisions or *cun.*

Acupuncture points by region

In Figures 19.4–19.13, we present the points by region. In the accompanying Tables 19.1.1 to 19.1.5 descriptions of the points are given, together with notes on locating them where relevant, and some conditions for which they are commonly. Also listed is the innervation of the dermatome (D), myotome (M) and sclerotome (S), where this information is relevant clinically. When the point's sclerotome is not applicable (e.g. because the periosteum is not accessible), no level is given. Where a point clearly relates to a single MTrP, the relevant muscle is named.

Needling direction can be assumed to be perpendicular unless stated otherwise.

The site of the MTrP is indicated with a cross-hatch symbol (rather than the usual X in other texts) so that the long strokes of the symbol indicate the muscle fibre orientation (Fig. 19.3). The two-tone shaded areas are examples of possible pain referral patterns from each MTrP, the darker areas indicating more common sites of pain.

An exclamation mark (!) against a point or directions for use indicates a particular risk. No needle should be inserted without first considering whether the local anatomy presents risks to treatment.

Clinical conditions for which the point is commonly used are listed (Figs 19.4–19.13).

Other reference tables

Table 19.2 shows segmental levels of the autonomic innervation of the body.

Table 19.3 shows spinal segmental levels and their relationship to acupuncture points.

Figure 19.14 shows the dermatomes of the back.

Table 19.4 shows some common sites for periosteal pecking that are accessible and generally safe.

Clinical observations suggest that the points shown in Table 19.5 are likely to be particularly useful for descending analgesic effects and central regulatory effects. They appear repeatedly in the formulae for treatment of a wide range of conditions, usually treated bilaterally.

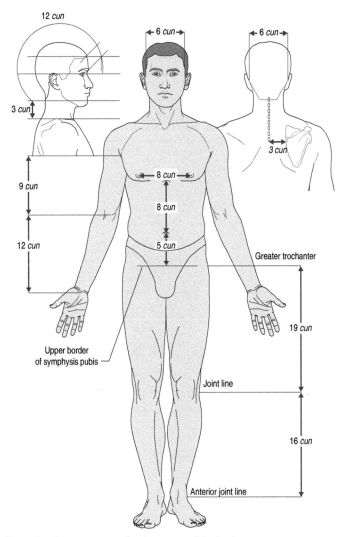

Figure 19.1 Proportional measurement of various parts of the body.

Since there is no evidence that the meridians have any physical structure or physiological function (apart from following palpable fascial planes in the upper arm), there seems little point in learning their pathways in detail. They can be useful insofar as they act as *aide-memoire* for the acupuncture points. Figures 19.15 and 19.16, and Tables 19.6 and 19.7 show what we think may be helpful or relevant to medical acupuncturists. Note that we present the meridians in the traditional order simply by convention.

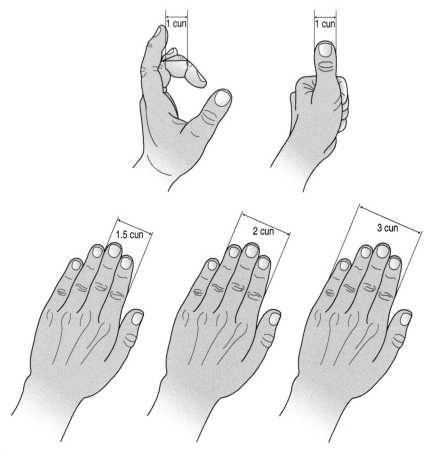

Figure 19.2 Use of the fingers and thumb to measure one, two and three cun.

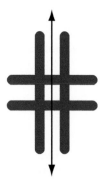

Figure 19.3 Cross-hatch symbol used to indicate the trigger point, the longitudinal strokes indicating the muscle fibre orientation.

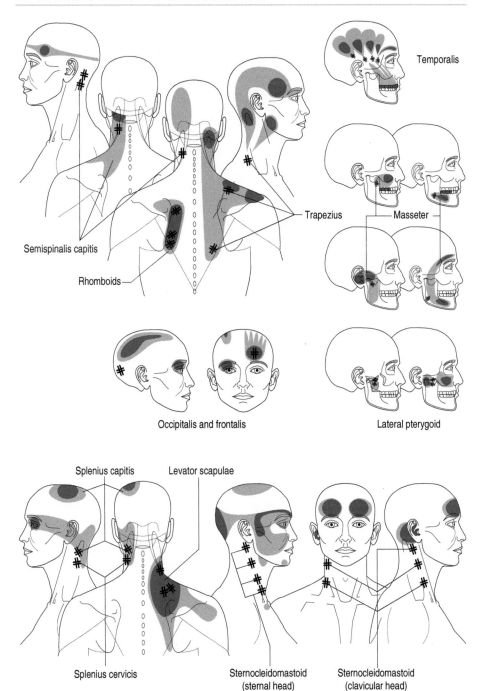

Figure 19.4 Head, face and neck: myofascial trigger points and pain reference zones.

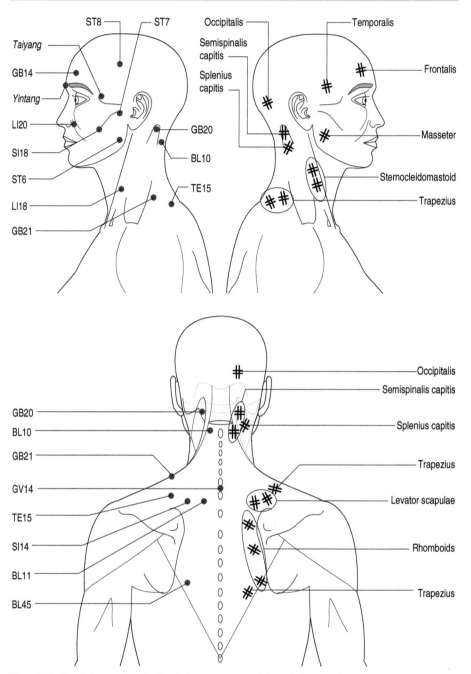

Figure 19.5 Head, face and neck: classical acupuncture points and trigger points.

TABLE 19.1.1 ▧ Head, neck and face

Head and neck

GB20	Below the occipital bone, in the depression between trapezius and sternomastoid and above splenius capitis **Angulation:** towards **Target:** semispinalis capitis opposite eyebrow *Headache, neck pain and stiffness* **CAUTION – note the position of the vertebral artery**	D C2/C3 M C1/C2 S C1/C2
BL10	1.3 *cun* lateral to the spinous process of C2, between C1 and C2 **Angulation:** towards **Target:** obliquus inferior lamina of C2 *Neck pain and stiffness* **CAUTION – note the position and depth of the spinal cord and vertebral artery**	D C3 M C1 to C5 S C2/C3
GB21	Midway between GV14 and tip of the acromion at the highest point of trapezius **Angulation:** tangential to **Target:** upper trapezius ribs, posteriorly *Headache, neck pain and stiffness, anxiety* **CAUTION – note the proximity of the pleura between the 1st and 2nd ribs**	D C3 M C3/C4 S n/a
TE15	Midway between the points GB21 and SI13 at the superior angle of the scapula (SI13 – tender depression superior to medial end of scapular spine) **Angulation:** perpendicular **Target:** trapezius *Shoulder pain, neck pain and stiffness* **CAUTION – note the proximity of the pleura in slim patients**	D C3 M C3/C4 S n/a
GV14	Between spinous processes C7 and T1 **Angulation:** transverse **Target:** interspinous ligament *Spinal neck pain, headache of cervical origin*	D C4/C5/T1 M C8 S C8
SI14	3 *cun* lateral to spinous process of T1 **Angulation:** tangential **Target:** levator scapulae towards scapula *Shoulder pain, neck pain and stiffness* **CAUTION – do not needle deeply unless confident of angulation relative to scapula**	D C3/C4 M C3/C4/C5 S C5
BL11	1.5 *cun* lateral to the lower border of the spinous process of T1 **Angulation:** oblique **Target:** rhomboid minor towards spine *Neck pain and stiffness, dyspnoea* **CAUTION – do not needle deeply unless confident of angulation relative to pleura**	D C4/T1 M C4/C5 S T1/T2
BL45	3 *cun* lateral to the lower border of the spinous process of T6 **Angulation:** oblique **Target:** iliocostalis thoracis towards spine *Dorsal back pain, dyspnoea* **CAUTION – do not needle deeply unless confident of angulation relative to pleura**	D T5/T6 M T6/T7 S T6/T7

Continued on following page

TABLE 19.1.1 ■ **Head, neck and face** (continued)

Face		
Yintang	Midpoint between the eyebrows **Angulation:** oblique **Target:** procerus or periosteum inferior *Headache, hayfever, relaxation*	D Vi M VII S Vi
Taiyang	1 *cun* posterior to the midpoint between the lateral end of the eyebrow and the lateral canthus of the eye **Angulation:** perpendicular **Target:** temporalis *Headache, eye symptoms*	D Vii M Viii S Vii
GB14	1 *cun* above the middle of the eyebrow, directly above the pupil when the eyes are looking straight ahead **Angulation:** oblique inferior **Target:** frontalis *Headache, eye symptoms*	D Vi M VII S Vi
LI 20	In the nasolabial groove, level with the widest part of the ala nasi **Angulation:** superiorly **Target:** facial muscles along groove *Hayfever, nasal symptoms*	D Vii M VII S Vii
ST6	1 fingerbreadth anterior and superior to the angle of the jaw, on the prominence of masseter **Angulation:** perpendicular **Target:** masseter *Dental pain, facial pain*	D C2/C3 M Viii S Viii
ST7	In the depression anterior to the temporomandibular joint and below the zygomatic arch **Angulation:** perpendicular **Target:** lateral pterygoid *Dental pain, facial pain*	D Viii M Viii S Viii
ST8	0.5 *cun* superior to the upper line of origin of the temporalis muscle, directly above ST7 and ST6 on a vertical line 0.5 cun posterior to Taiyang **Angulation:** perpendicular **Target:** epicranial tissues *Headache*	D Vi/Vii M Viii/VII S Vi/Vii
SI18	Directly below the lateral canthus of the eye in the depression at the lower border of the zygomatic bone, just anterior to the attachment of masseter **Angulation:** slightly superior **Target:** connective tissue space *Facial pain, trigeminal neuralgia*	D Vii M Viii S Vii
LI18	Between the sternal and clavicular heads of sternocleidomastoid (SCM), level with the laryngeal prominence (the tip of the Adam's apple) **Angulation:** posterior **Target:** fascial plane in SCM *Pain from sternocleidomastoid – headache or facial pain* **CAUTION – note the proximity of the carotid artery**	D C2/C3 M XI/C2/C3 S n/a

D = dermatome, M = myotome, S = sclerotome, V = trigeminal nerve, i = ophthalmic, ii = maxillary, iii =
mandibular divisions, VII = facial nerve, XI = accessory nerve, n/a = not applicable
Meridian abbreviations – see Tables 19.6 and 19.7, page 211.

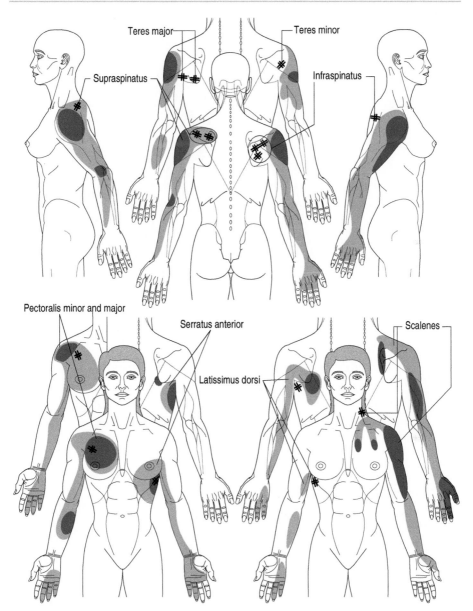

Figure 19.6   Shoulder and arm: myofascial trigger points and pain reference zones.

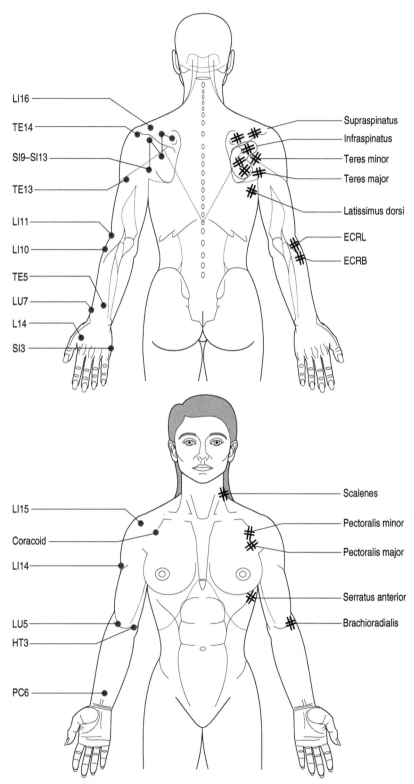

Figure 19.7 Shoulder and arm: classical acupuncture points and trigger points.

TABLE 19.1.2 ■ Shoulder and arm

Posterior aspect

LI16	In the depression medial to the acromion and between the lateral extremities of the clavicle and scapular spine **Angulation:** perpendicular **Target:** supraspinatus *Shoulder and arm pain*	D C3 M C3–C6 S C5/C6
TE14	Posterolateral and inferior to the posterior tip of the acromion, in the depression between the middle and posterior fibres of deltoid **Angulation:** perpendicular **Target:** infraspinatus insertion *Shoulder and arm pain*	D C3/C4 M C5/C6 S C6
SI9	1 *cun* superior to the posterior axillary crease when the arm hangs by the side of the body **Angulation:** perpendicular **Target:** teres major *Shoulder and arm pain*	D T3/T4 M C5/C6/C7 S C7
SI10	In the depression below the spine of the scapula, directly superior to the posterior axillary crease when the arm hangs by the side of the body **Angulation:** perpendicular **Target:** infraspinatus *Shoulder and arm pain*	D C3/C4 M C5/C6 S C6
SI11	One-third down a line from the midpoint of the scapular spine to the inferior angle of the scapula **Angulation:** perpendicular **Target:** infraspinatus *Shoulder and arm pain*	D C4/T1/T2 M C5/C6 S C5/C6
SI12	Directly above SI11 in the middle of the suprascapular fossa, about 1 *cun* above the middle of the superior border of the scapular spine **Angulation:** towards suprascapular fossa *Shoulder and arm pain* **CAUTION – do not needle deeply unless confident of position relative to scapula**	D C3/C4 M C3–C6 S C5
SI13	In the tender depression superior to the medial end of the scapular spine **Angulation:** towards suprascapular fossa *Shoulder and arm pain* **CAUTION – do not needle deeply unless confident of position relative to scapula**	D C4/T1 M C3–C6 S C5
TE13	On the line connecting the olecranon and TE14, 3 cun distal to TE14 on the posterior border of deltoid, 2 cun lateral to the posterior axillary fold **Angulation:** perpendicular **Target:** lateral head of triceps *Shoulder and arm pain* **CAUTION – note the proximity of the radial nerve**	D C5 M C6/C7/C8 S C6/C7
LI11	At the radial end of the antecubital crease, halfway between the biceps tendon and the lateral epicondyle **Angulation:** perpendicular **Target:** extensor carpi radialis longus *Lateral epicondylalgia, forearm pain; immunomodulation*	D C5/C6 M C5/C6 S C6/C7
LI10	2 *cun* distal to LI11, on the line connecting LI11 with LI5 (the centre of the anatomical snuff box) **Angulation:** perpendicular **Target:** extensor carpi radialis longus or supinator *Lateral epicondylalgia, forearm pain*	D C5/C6 M C5/C6/C7 S C6/C7

Continued on following page

TABLE 19.1.2 ■ **Shoulder and arm** (continued)

Posterior aspect

TE5	On the dorsal surface of forearm, 2 *cun* proximal to wrist joint, between radius and ulna, and between extensor indicis and extensor pollicis longus **Angulation:** perpendicular **Target:** connective tissue plane *Local pain; wrist and forearm; major point for central effects*	D C6–C8 M C7/C8 S C7/C8
LU7	On the radial aspect of the radial styloid, 1.5 *cun* from the wrist crease, between the tendons of abductor pollicis longus and brachioradialis **Angulation:** proximal oblique **Target:** connective tissue space *Wrist and forearm pain*	D C6 M C7/C8 S C6
LI4	On the dorsal aspect of the hand, in the middle of the 1st web space, halfway along the second metacarpal bone **Angulation:** perpendicular **Target:** 1st dorsal interosseous *General point for pain; major point for central effects* **CAUTION – the radial artery is at the apex of the 1st web space**	D C6/C7 M T1 S n/a
SI3	On the palmar aspect of the neck of the 5th metacarpal, in the tissue plane between the metacarpal neck and the hypothenar muscles **Angulation:** perpendicular **Target:** connective tissue plane *Hand pain; also used for pain elsewhere, especially spinal pain*	D C8 M T1 S C8

Anterior aspect

LI15	Anterolateral and inferior to the anterior tip of the acromion, in the groove between the anterior and middle fibres of deltoid **Angulation:** perpendicular **Target:** supraspinatus insertion *Shoulder and arm pain*	D C4 M C5 S C5
Coracoid	Anterior to the glenohumeral joint, between the fibres of deltoid and pectoralis major **Angulation:** perpendicular **Target:** coracoid *Shoulder and arm pain*	D C4 M C5/C6 S C5
LI14	Between the distal attachment of deltoid and the long head of biceps, in a tender depression, 3/5 of the distance on a line from LI11–LI15 **Angulation:** perpendicular **Target:** connective tissue plane *Shoulder and arm pain*	D C5/C6 M C5/C6 S C5/C6
LU5	On the cubital crease of the elbow, in the depression on the radial side of the biceps tendon **Angulation:** perpendicular **Target:** brachioradialis *Elbow or forearm pain*	D C5/C6 M C5/C6 S C5/C6
HT3	At the medial end of the antecubital crease when the elbow is fully flexed **Angulation:** perpendicular **Target:** pronator teres *Medial epicondylalgia, forearm pain* **CAUTION – note the proximity of the brachial artery**	D T1 M C5–T1 S C7
PC6	2 *cun* proximal to the distal wrist crease, between the tendons of flexor carpi radialis and palmaris longus **Angulation:** oblique proximal **Target:** flexor digitorum superficialis *Nausea and vomiting, carpal tunnel syndrome* **CAUTION – note the position of the median nerve directly below**	D C6/C8/T1 M C7/C8 S n/a

D = dermatome, M = myotome, S = sclerotome, V = trigeminal nerve, i = ophthalmic, ii = maxillary, iii = mandibular divisions, VII = facial nerve, XI = accessory nerve, n/a = not applicable
Meridian abbreviations – see Tables 19.6 and 19.7, page 211.

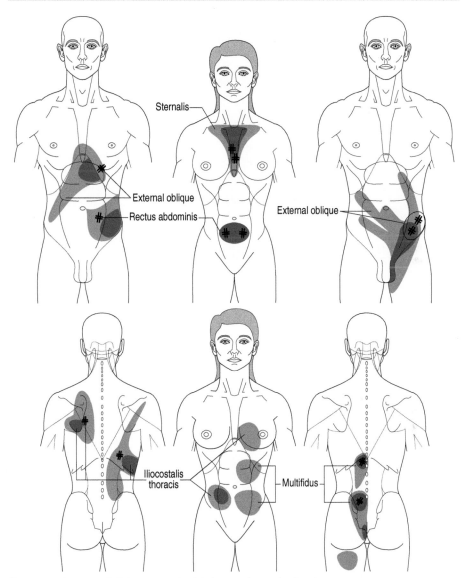

Figure 19.8 Thorax and abdomen: myofascial trigger points and pain reference zones.

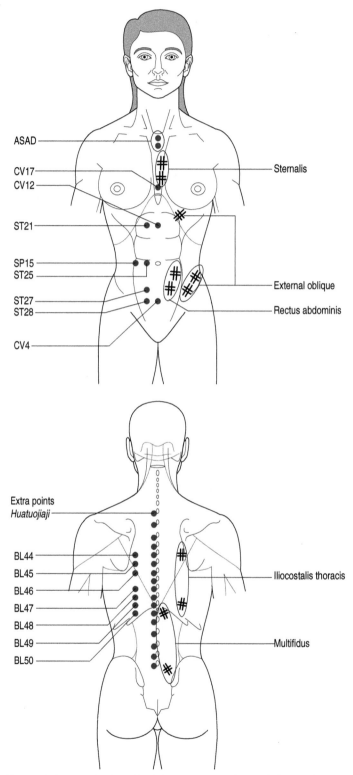

Figure 19.9 Thorax, abdomen and spine: classical acupuncture points and trigger points.

TABLE 19.1.3 ■ **Thorax and abdomen**

Anterior aspect			
ASAD	Two points in the midline just below the sternal notch over the manubrium		D C4/T2 M C5/C6
	Angulation: perpendicular	**Target:** periosteum of manubrium	S T1
	Anxiety, sickness and dyspnoea		
CV17	In the centre of the sternum at the 4th intercostal space (level with nipples in a man)		D T5 M C8, T1
	Angulation: cranial oblique at 30 degrees to the sternum	**Target:** periosteum of the sternum or sternalis	S T1
	Chest pain; respiratory conditions		
	CAUTION – a sternal foramen occurs at this point in 10% of men and 4% of women; never needle perpendicularly		
CV12	On the midline of the upper abdomen, midway between the umbilicus and the lower border of the body of the sternum		D T8 M T8
	Angulation: perpendicular	**Target:** linea alba	S n/a
	Upper gastrointestinal disorders, including nausea and vomiting		
	CAUTION – avoid needling through the abdominal wall		
CV4	On the midline of the lower abdomen, 3 *cun* inferior to the umbilicus and 2 *cun* superior to the pubic symphysis		D T11/T12 M T11/T12
	Angulation: perpendicular	**Target:** linea alba	S n/a
	Lower *gastrointestinal, urological and gynaecological symptoms*		
	CAUTION – avoid needling through the abdominal wall		
SP15	At the lateral border of rectus abdominis level with the umbilicus		D T10/T11 M T10/T11
	Angulation: perpendicular	**Target:** linea semilunaris	S n/a
	Abdominal pain		
	CAUTION – avoid needling through the abdominal wall		

Kidney and Stomach meridians run parallel with CV, with points over the abdomen at most segments – any tender point can be treated

ST21	2 *cun* lateral to CV12		D T7/T8 M T7/T8
	Angulation: medial oblique [non-classical]	**Target:** rectus abdominis	S n/a
	Upper abdominal pain; gastroenterological symptoms		
	CAUTION – avoid needling through the abdominal wall		
ST25	2 *cun* lateral to the umbilicus, halfway between the umbilicus and the linea semilunaris (SP15)		D T10 M T10
	Angulation: perpendicular	**Target:** rectus abdominis	S n/a
	Abdominal pain; gastroenterological symptoms		
	CAUTION – avoid needling through the abdominal wall		
ST27	2 *cun* lateral to the midline and 2 *cun* inferior to the umbilicus		D T11/T12 M T11/T12
	Angulation: medial oblique [non-classical]	**Target:** rectus abdominis	S n/a
	Abdominal pain; lower gastrointestinal, urological and gynaecological symptoms		
	CAUTION – avoid needling through the abdominal wall		

Continued on following page

TABLE 19.1.3 ■ **Thorax and abdomen** (continued)

Anterior aspect

ST28	2 *cun* lateral to the midline and 3 *cun* inferior to the umbilicus **Angulation:** medial oblique **Target:** rectus abdominis [non-classical] *Abdominal pain; lower gastrointestinal, urological and* *gynaecological symptoms* **CAUTION – avoid needling through the abdominal wall**	D T12/L1 M T12/L1 S n/a

Posterior aspect

Huatuojiaji	A series of 17 extra points, 0.5 *cun* lateral to the lower border of the spinous processes of T1 to L5 **Angulation:** oblique towards spine **Target:** multifidus *Spinal pain; segmental acupuncture*	D T1–L1 M T1–L5 S T1–L5
Bladder line *– outer*	3 *cun* lateral to the midline, on a vertical line joining the medial edge of the scapula and the outer border of the lumbar erector spinae **Angulation:** oblique towards spine **Target:** iliocostalis thoracis *Dorsal back pain, ventral pain* **CAUTION – do not needle deeply unless confident of** **angulation relative to pleura**	D T5–T9 M T6–T12 S T6–T12 – rib level
BL44	Level with the lower border of T5	
BL45	Level with the lower border of T6	
BL46	Level with the lower border of T7	
BL47	Level with the lower border of T9	
BL48	Level with the lower border of T10	
BL49	Level with the lower border of T11	
BL50	Level with the lower border of T12	

D = dermatome, M = myotome, S = sclerotome, V = trigeminal nerve, i = ophthalmic, ii = maxillary,
    iii?=?mandibular divisions, VII = facial nerve, XI?=?accessory nerve, n/a = not applicable
Meridian abbreviations – see Tables 19.6 and 19.7, page 211.

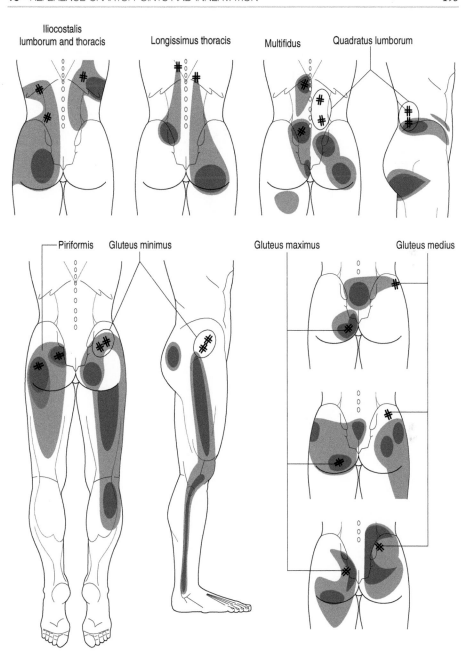

Figure 19.10   Low back and hip girdle: myofascial trigger points and pain reference zones.

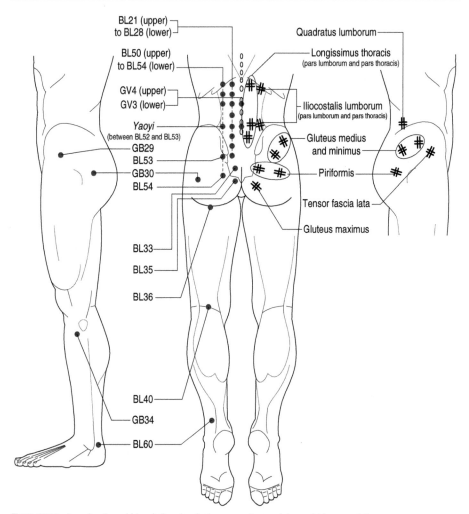

Figure 19.11   Low back and hip girdle: classical acupuncture points and trigger points.

TABLE 19.1.4 ■ Back and hip girdle

Lateral aspect

GB29	Midway between the anterior superior iliac spine and the greater trochanter **Angulation:** perpendicular **Target:** tensor fasciae latae *Hip girdle pain* **CAUTION – deep needling may penetrate the capsule of the hip joint**	D L2/L3 M L5/S1/S2 S L4/L5/S1
GB30	One-third of the way from the highest point of the greater trochanter to the sacral hiatus **Angulation:** towards symphysis **Target:** tensor fasciae latae pubis *Hip girdle pain, back pain, leg pain, sciatica* **CAUTION – avoid direct needling of the sciatic nerve**	D L2/L3 M L5/S1/S2 S L4/L5/S1
GB34	In the depression just anterior and inferior to the head of the fibula **Angulation:** perpendicular **Target:** peroneus longus *Leg pain; general point for musculoskeletal pain* **CAUTION – avoid needling the common fibular nerve**	D L5 M L5/S1 S L5
BL60	In the depression midway between the lateral malleolus and the Achilles tendon **Angulation:** perpendicular **Target:** connective tissue *Leg pain, Achilles tendon pain*	D L5/S1 M L5/S1 S S1/S2

Posterior aspect

GV4	Between spinous processes L2 and L3 **Angulation:** transverse **Target:** interspinous ligament *Spinal pain*	D T9/T10 M L2 S L2
GV3	Between spinous processes L4 and L5 **Angulation:** transverse **Target:** interspinous ligament *Spinal pain*	D T11/T12 M L4 S L4
Huatuo-jiaji	A series of 17 extra points, 0.5 *cun* lateral to the lower border of the spinous processes of T1 to L5 **Angulation:** oblique towards spine **Target:** multifidus *Spinal pain; segmental acupuncture*	D T1–L1 M T1–L5 S T1–L5
BL line – inner	1.5 *cun* lateral to the midline, halfway between the Outer Bladder line and the spine **Angulation:** oblique towards spine **Target:** erector spinae *Back pain*	D T9–S2 S T12–S2
BL21	Level with the lower border of T12	M T10/T11
BL22	Level with the lower border of L1	M T11/T12
BL23	Level with the lower border of L2	M T12/L1
BL24	Level with the lower border of L3	M L1/L2
BL25	Level with the lower border of L4	M L2/L3
BL26	Level with the lower border of L5	M L3/L4
BL27	Level with the S1 posterior foramen, or upper aspect of the posterior superior iliac spine **Angulation:** perpendicular **Target:** erector spinae or multifidus	M L4 S S1

Continued on following page

TABLE 19.1.4 ■ **Back and hip girdle** (continued)

Posterior aspect		
BL28	Level with the S2 posterior foramen, or the lower aspect of the posterior superior iliac spine **Angulation:** perpendicular　　　　**Target:** erector spinae or multifidus	M L5 S S2
BL33	Over the S3 posterior foramen **Angulation:** perpendicular　　　　**Target:** S3 posterior foramen *Local pain; disturbance of pelvic organs (e.g. detrusor instability)*	D S2/S3 M L5 S S3
BL35	0.5 *cun* lateral to the tip of the coccyx **Angulation:** perpendicular　　　　**Target:** sacrotuberous ligament *Coccydinia*	D S3/S4 M L5/S1/S2 S S4/ coccygeal
BL36	In the transverse gluteal crease, in a depression between the hamstring muscles **Angulation:** perpendicular　　　　**Target:** hamstring attachment *Local pain, hamstring pain, sciatica*	D S2/S3 M L5/S1/S2 S L5
BL40	On the popliteal crease midway between the tendons of biceps femoris and semitendinosus **Angulation:** perpendicular　　　　**Target:** connective tissue *Local pain, sciatica*	D S1/S2 M S1/S2 S n/a
BL line – outer	3 *cun* lateral to the midline, on a vertical line joining the medial edge of the scapula and the outer border of the lumbar erector spinae **Angulation:** oblique towards spine unless stated otherwise below *Back pain*	D T9–S2 S n/a mostly
BL50	Level with the lower border of T12	M T10/T11
BL51	Level with the lower border of L1	M T11/T12
BL52	Level with the lower border of L2	M T12/L1
Yaoyi	Level with the lower border of L4	M L2/L3
BL53	Level with the S2 posterior foramen, or the lower aspect of the posterior superior iliac spine **Angulation:** perpendicular　　　　**Target:** gluteus medius *Hip girdle pain, back pain*	D L2/S3 M L4–S2 S L5
BL54	Level with the S4 posterior foramen in the sciatic notch **Angulation:** perpendicular　　　　**Target:** piriformis *Hip girdle pain, back pain, leg pain, sciatica* **CAUTION – avoid needling the sciatic nerve**	D S2/S3 M L5–S2 S S2/S3
BL60	At the level of the most prominent part of the lateral malleolus, halfway between it and the Achilles tendon **Angulation:** perpendicular　　　　**Target:** connective tissue space *Painful conditions, especially of spine, distant point in sciatica*	D L5/S1 M L5/S1 S n/a

D = dermatome, M = myotome, S = sclerotome, V = trigeminal nerve, i = ophthalmic, ii = maxillary, iii = mandibular divisions, VII = facial nerve, XI = accessory nerve, n/a = not applicable
Meridian abbreviations – see Tables 19.6 and 19.7, page 211.

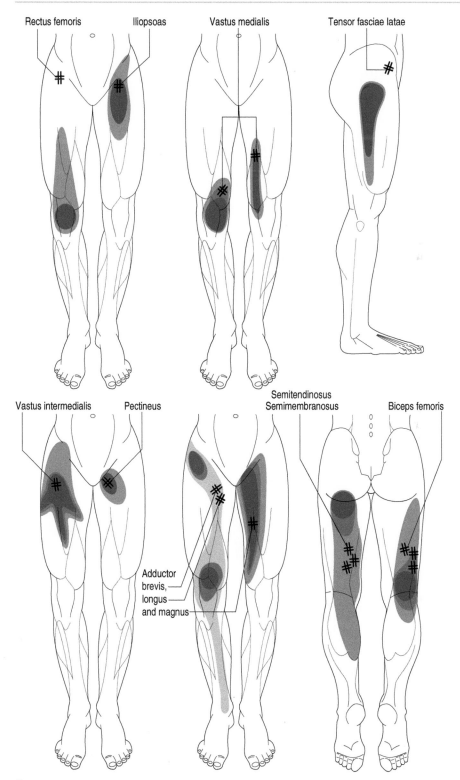

Figure 19.12 Lower limb: myofascial trigger points and pain reference zones.

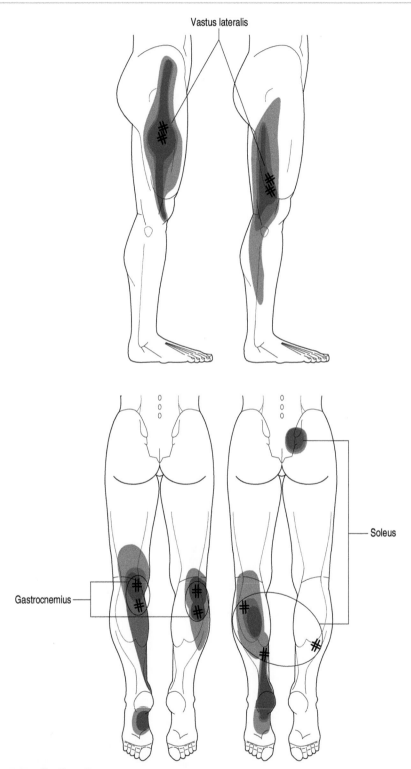

Figure 19.12 *Continued*

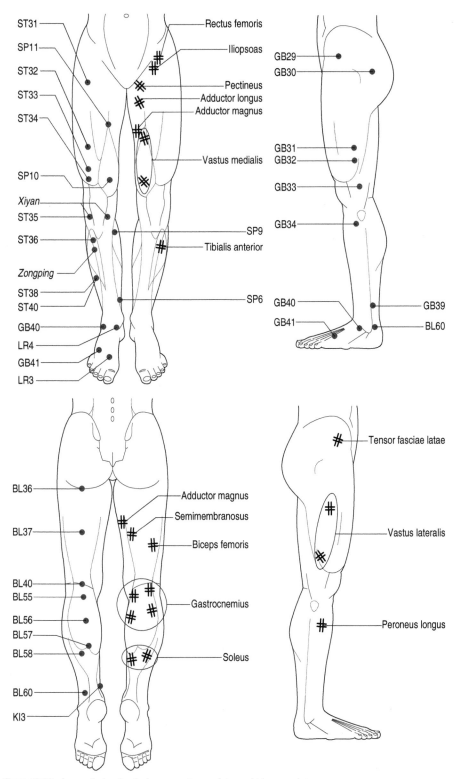

Figure 19.13 Lower limb: classical acupuncture points and trigger points.

TABLE 19.1.5 ▪ Lower limb

Thigh and lower leg: anterior aspect

ST31	In a depression just lateral to sartorius, at the junction of a vertical line through the anterior superior iliac spine and a horizontal line at the level of the lower border of the pubic symphysis **Angulation:** perpendicular **Target:** rectus femoris *Thigh pain, anterior knee pain (rectus femoris)*	D L2 M L2/L3/L4 S L3/L4
ST32	6 *cun* superior to the upper lateral margin of the patella on a line that joins the lateral border of the patella to the anterior superior iliac spine **Angulation:** perpendicular **Target:** vastus lateralis *Thigh pain*	D L2 M L3/L4 S L3
ST33	3 *cun* superior to the upper lateral margin of the patella on a line that joins the lateral border of the patella to the anterior superior iliac spine **Angulation:** perpendicular **Target:** vastus lateralis *Thigh and knee pain*	D L2/L3 M L3/L4 S L3
ST34	2 *cun* superior to the upper lateral margin of the patella on a line that joins the lateral border of the patella to the anterior superior iliac spine **Angulation:** perpendicular **Target:** vastus lateralis *Knee pain*	D L2/L3 M L3/L4 S L3
ST35	In the hollow on the lateral aspect of the patella tendon directly over the joint line **Angulation:** towards the patella **Target:** knee capsule tendon [non-classical] *Knee pain* **CAUTION – avoid needling into the knee joint**	D L3/L4/L5 M L3/L4 S L3/L4/L5
Xiyan	In the hollows on either side of the patella tendon directly over the joint line **Angulation:** towards the patella **Target:** knee capsule tendon [non-classical] *Knee pain* **CAUTION – avoid needling into the knee joint**	D L3/L4/L5 M L3/L4 S L3/L4/L5
ST36	3 *cun* inferior to the knee joint, 1 fingerbreadth lateral to the lower border of the tibial tuberosity, in the middle of the upper third of the tibialis anterior **Angulation:** perpendicular **Target:** tibialis anterior *Knee pain, abdominal problems, major combination for central effects*	D L4/L5 M L4/L5 S L4/L5
Zongping	1 *cun* inferior to ST36 **Angulation:** perpendicular **Target:** tibialis anterior *Used with ST36 for EA – major combination for central effects*	D L4/L5 M L4/L5 S L4/L5
ST40	On the anterolateral aspect of the lower leg, midway between the tibiofemoral joint line and the lateral malleolus, 2 fingerbreadths lateral to the anterior crest of the tibia **Angulation:** perpendicular **Target:** extensor hallucis longus *Local pain; a variety of traditional indications* **CAUTION – avoid needling to the depth of the anterior tibial artery**	D L5 M L5/S1 S L5/S1
SP11	6 *cun* superior to SP10, on a line connecting SP10 with SP12 **Angulation:** perpendicular **Target:** vastus medialis *Thigh and knee pain (vastus medialis)* **CAUTION – note the position of the femoral artery**	D L3 M L2/L3/L4 S L3

TABLE 19.1.5 ■ **Lower limb** (continued)

Thigh and lower leg: anterior aspect

SP10	2 *cun* proximal to the superiomedial border of the patella, in the centre of vastus medialis **Angulation:** perpendicular **Target:** vastus medialis *Knee pain (vastus medialis)*	D L3 M L2/L3/L4 S L3
SP9	In a depression inferior to the medial condyle of the tibia and posterior to the medial border of the tibia, at the same level as GB34 **Angulation:** perpendicular **Target:** connective tissue space *Knee pain, gynaecological and urological problems*	D L3 M L2/L3/L4 S L3
SP6	3 *cun* superior to the most prominent part of the medial malleolus, on the medial border of the tibia **Angulation:** perpendicular **Target:** flexor digitorum longus *Gynaecological problems; major point for central effects*	D L4/S1/S2 M S1/S2 S L4/L5
LR4	Anterior to the medial malleolus, in the depression just medial to the tendon of tibialis anterior **Angulation:** perpendicular **Target:** connective tissue space *Ankle pain* **CAUTION – avoid needling into the ankle joint**	D L4/L5 M L4/L5 S L4/L5
LR3	On the dorsum of the foot, in the 1st metatarsal space, in a depression distal to the junction of the bases of the 1st and 2nd metatarsals **Angulation:** perpendicular **Target:** 1st dorsal interosseous *Local pain; headache; abdominal problems; major point for central effects* **CAUTION – the dorsalis pedis artery is at the apex of the 1st metatarsal space**	D L4/L5 M S2/S3 S L5/S1

Thigh and lower leg: lateral aspect

GB29	On the lateral aspect of the hip midway between the anterior superior iliac spine and the greater trochanter **Angulation:** perpendicular **Target:** tensor fasciae latae or glutei *Hip girdle pain* **CAUTION – deep needling may penetrate the capsule of the hip joint**	D L2 M L4/L5/S1 S L3/L4/L5
GB30	One-third of the way to the sacral hiatus from the most prominent part of the greater trochanter **Angulation:** perpendicular **Target:** lateral piriformis *Low back pain, hip girdle pain, sciatica* **CAUTION – avoid needling the sciatic nerve**	D L2/L3/S2 M L5/S1/S2 S L4/L5/S1
GB31	7 *cun* above the popliteal crease in the palpable furrow just posterior to the iliotibial tract **Angulation:** perpendicular **Target:** vastus lateralis or intermedius *Thigh and knee pain*	D L2 M L3/L4 S L3

Continued on following page

TABLE 19.1.5 ■ **Lower limb** (continued)

Thigh and lower leg: lateral aspect

GB32	In the palpable furrow just posterior to the iliotibial tract, 2 *cun* below GB32	D L2 M L3/L4
	Angulation: perpendicular · · · · · **Target:** vastus lateralis or intermedius	S L3
	Thigh and knee pain	
GB33	On the lateral aspect of the knee 3 *cun* superior to GB34, in a depression between the femur and the tendon of biceps femoris	D L2/L3/S2 M L4 to S2
	Angulation: perpendicular · · · · · **Target:** connective tissue space	S L3/L4
	Knee pain	
	CAUTION – if the knee is flexed this point is close to the posterior joint margin	
GB34	In the depression about 1 *cun* anterior and inferior to the head of the fibula	D L5 M L5/S1
	Angulation: perpendicular · · · · · **Target:** peroneus longus	S L5
	Knee pain	
	CAUTION – avoid deep needling since the anterior tibial artery and common fibular nerve are deep to this point	
GB39	3 *cun* superior to the lateral malleolus, between the fibular shaft and the tendon of peroneus longus (use digital pressure to form a groove between the tendon and the fibula)	D L5/S1 M L5/S1
	Angulation: perpendicular · · · · · **Target:** peroneus brevis	S L5/S1
	Lower leg and ankle pain	
	CAUTION – avoid forceful ankle movement when a needle is placed in this point	
GB40	In the depression anterior and inferior to the lateral malleolus	D L5/S1 M L5/S1
	Angulation: perpendicular · · · · · **Target:** connective tissue space	S S1/S2
	Ankle pain	
	CAUTION – avoid needling into the ankle joint	
GB41	In the depression distal to the junction of the 4th and 5th metatarsals, lateral to the tendon of extensor digitorum longus that passes to the 5th toe	D L5/S1 M S1/S2 S S2
	Angulation: perpendicular · · · · · **Target:** 4th dorsal interosseous	
	Forefoot pain	

Thigh and lower leg – posterior aspect

BL36	In the transverse gluteal crease, in a depression between the hamstring muscles	D S2/S3 M L5/S1/S2
	Angulation: perpendicular · · · · · **Target:** hamstring attachment	S L5
	Local pain, hamstring pain, sciatica	
BL40	On the popliteal crease midway between the tendons of biceps femoris and semitendinosus, in the connective tissue space between the heads of gastrocnemius	D S1/S2 M S1/S2
	Angulation: perpendicular · · · · · **Target:** connective tissue space	S n/a
	Local pain, sciatica	
	CAUTION – note the popliteal artery and tibial nerve are deep to this point	

TABLE 19.1.5 ▪ **Lower limb** (continued)

Thigh and lower leg – posterior aspect

BL55	2 *cun* inferior to BL40, on the line connecting BL40 and BL57, between the two heads of gastrocnemius	D S1/S2 M S1/S2
	Angulation: perpendicular　　　　**Target:** fascial plane *Calf pain*	S n/a
BL56	In the fascial plane between the heads of gastrocnemius, 5 *cun* below BL40, midway between BL55 and BL57	D S1/S2 M S1/S2
	Angulation: perpendicular　　　　**Target:** fascial plane *Calf pain*	S n/a
BL57	In the depression formed below the bellies of the gastrocnemius muscle when the muscle is flexed, midway between BL40 and BL60	D S1/S2 M S1/S2
	Angulation: perpendicular　　　　**Target:** musculotendinous junction *Calf pain*	S n/a
BL58	7 *cun* directly superior to BL60, lateral to and approximately 1 *cun* inferior to BL57, at the musculotendinous junction of the lateral head of gastrocnemius	D L5/S1/S2 M S1/S2 S n/a
	Angulation: perpendicular　　　　**Target:** musculotendinous junction *Calf pain*	
BL60	At the level of the most prominent part of the lateral malleolus, halfway between it and the Achilles tendon	D L5/S1 M L5/S1
	Angulation: perpendicular　　　　**Target:** connective tissue space *Painful conditions, especially of spine, distant point in sciatica*	S n/a
KI3	At the level of the most prominent part of the medial malleolus, halfway between it and the Achilles tendon	D L4/S2 M S2
	Angulation: perpendicular　　　　**Target:** connective tissue space *Ankle problems; urogenital problems; major point for central effects*	S n/a

D = dermatome, M = myotome, S = sclerotome, V = trigeminal nerve, i = ophthalmic, ii = maxillary, iii = mandibular divisions, VII = facial nerve, XI = accessory nerve, n/a = not applicable
Meridian abbreviations – see Tables 19.6 and 19.7, page 211.

TABLE 19.2 ■ Segmental levels of the autonomic innervation of the body

Part or organ of body	Sympathetic	Parasympathetic
Head and neck	T1 to T5	Four cranial nerves
Upper limb	T2 to T9	Nil
Lower limb	T10 to L2	Nil
Heart	T1 to T5	Vagus
Lung and bronchi	T2 to T4	Vagus
Oesophagus (caudal part)	T5 to T6	Vagus
Stomach	T6 to T10	Vagus
Small intestine	T9 to T10	Vagus
Large intestine: to splenic flexure	T11 to L1	Vagus
Large intestine: splenic flexure to rectum	L1 to L2	S2 to S4
Liver and gall bladder	T7 to T9	Vagus
Testis and ovary	T10 to T11	Nil
Urinary bladder	T11 to L2	S2 to S4
Uterus	T12 to L1	S2 to S4

TABLE 19.3 ■ Spinal segmental levels and their relationship to acupuncture points

Region	Level	Dermatome	Myotome	Sclerotome[a]
Thoracic	1	GV14	LI4, SI3	
	2 to 8	see Fig. 19.14	*Huatuojiaji* point at each level	
	9	GV4		
	10	GV4, BL23, ST25	ST25	
	11	BL23, BL25, GV3, CV4	CV4	
	12	BL25, GV3, CV4	BL23, CzV4	
Lumbar	1		BL23	
	2		BL23, BL25, GV4, SP10	BL23, GV4
	3	SP9, L3	BL25, SP10 ·	SP9
	4	ST36, SP6, SP9, KI3, LR3	BL25, ST36, SP10	BL25, ST36, SP6, SP9, KI3, GV3
	5	ST36, LR3	ST36, BL54(49)	ST36, LR3
Sacral	1	SP6, BL40(54)	SP6, SP9, KI3	LR3
	2	SP6, KI3, BL40(54)	SP6, SP9, KI3, LR3	KI3
	3	BL54(49)		
	4			
	5			

[a]Sclerotomal points include the spinous process at each vertebral level; and bony promontories near the classical point given in this table, e.g. for KI3, the medial malleolus.

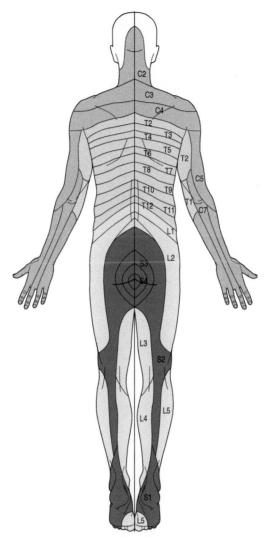

Figure 19.14 Dermatomes of the back. *(Reproduced with permission from Moffat DB, 1993. Lecture Notes on Anatomy, 2nd edn. John Wiley & Sons.)*

TABLE 19.4 ■ **Innervation of some sites used for periosteal pecking**

Target site for needling	Sclerotome
Occiput	C1
Acromion	C4
Spine of scapula	C4, C5
Greater tubercle of humerus	C5
Lateral epicondyle	C6, C7
Spinous process	Level of segment above (processes tend to angle inferiorly)
Iliac crest	L2
Greater trochanter	L5
Medial aspect of tibial plateau	L3, L4

TABLE 19.5 ■ **List of traditional points commonly regarded as 'major' points**

Limb	Major points
Arm	LI11
	LI4
	TE5
	PC6
Leg	ST36
	SP6
	LR3
	KI3

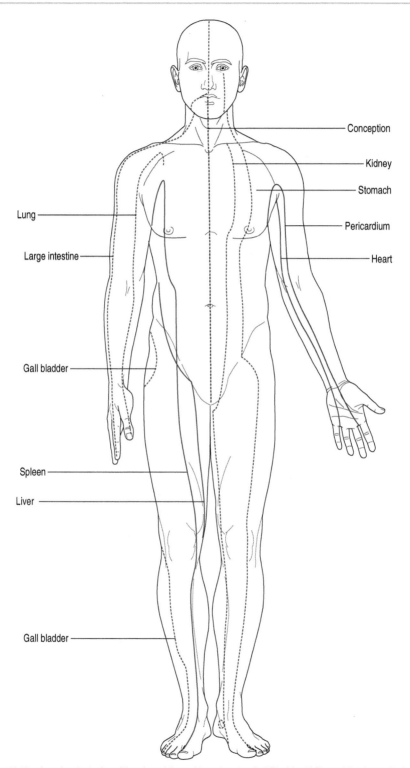

Figure 19.15 Anterior view of traditional meridians. Note that the Gall Bladder (GB) meridian is on the lateral surface and sections appear in each diagram.

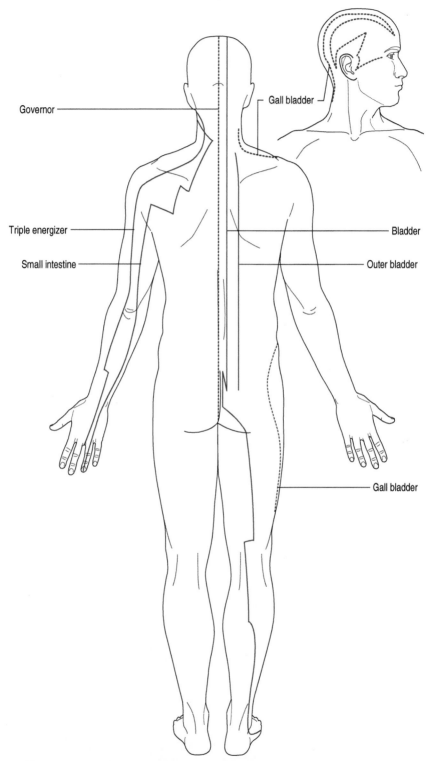

Figure 19.16 Posterior view of traditional meridians. Note that the Gall Bladder (GB) meridian is on the lateral surface and sections appear in each diagram.

TABLE 19.6 ■ **Meridians on the anterior surface of the body, their relevance to medical acupuncture, and alternative abbreviations**

Meridian name (and abbreviation)	Significance of the meridian in medical acupuncture	Alternative abbreviations in other texts[a]
Lung (LU)	Little relevance	L, P
Pericardium (PC)	Relevant only in PC6	HC, Pe
Heart (HT)	Little relevance	C, He
Stomach (ST)	Useful on the abdomen and again around the knee	E, M
Spleen (SP)	Only relevant at points at the ankle and knee	LP, RP
Kidney (KI)	Little relevance, occasionally the abdomen points are useful	K, R, Rn
Liver (LR)	Relevant only at LR3	Liv, H, Lv
Conception Vessel (CV)	Midline points that are relevant in both thorax and abdomen	Co, J, REN, VC

[a]Some abbreviations derive from names with Latin or French origin.

TABLE 19.7 ■ **Meridians on the posterior surface of the body, their relevance to medical acupuncture, and alternative abbreviations**

Meridian name (and abbreviation)	Significance of the meridian in medical acupuncture	Alternative abbreviations in other texts[a]
Large Intestine (LI)	Points are used at hand, elbow and shoulder and again at the final point near the nose	Co, IC
Triple Energizer (TE)	Relevant only in TE5	T, TB, TH, TW, SJ
Small Intestine (SI)	We meet this point at the medial border of the hand and more points around the scapula	IT
Gall Bladder (GB)	Points are used around the neck and shoulder. Other points in the head, and in the leg, will also be useful	G, VB, VF
Bladder (BL)	A long meridian, and points are commonly used especially down the paraspinal region and in the ankle	B, UB, VU
Governor Vessel (GV)	Midline points are used in the lower and upper spine	DU, Go, TM, VG

[a]Some abbreviations derive from names with Latin or French origin.

Further reading

Baldry, P.E., 2005. Acupuncture, Trigger Points and Musculoskeletal Pain. Elsevier, Edinburgh.

The illustrations and figures in this book will be particularly useful to acupuncturists who want to develop their knowledge and skill in treating myofascial pain.

Campbell, A., 2001. Acupuncture in Practice: Beyond Points and Meridians. Butterworth-Heinemann, Oxford.

Anthony Campbell describes a rational approach to treatment that he has developed from the traditional practice, using 'acupuncture treatment areas'. This book explains how to apply this approach throughout the body.

Hecker, H.U., Steveling, A., Peuker, E., et al., 2001. Color Atlas of Acupuncture. Thieme, Stuttgart.

This book is a model of clarity for anyone who wants exact descriptions of a selection of acupuncture points. However, it is full of traditional Chinese theory! It includes sections on body points, auricular points and myofascial trigger points.

Mann, F., 1992. Reinventing Acupuncture. Butterworth-Heinemann, Oxford.

Felix Mann describes his approach to treatment in detail, which is based on his observations and anatomical knowledge. He uses treatment areas rather than traditional points, and his approach is based on clinical experience not physiological mechanisms.

References

Allen, J.J.B., Schnyer, R.N., Hitt, S.K., 1998. The efficacy of acupuncture in the treatment of major depression in women. Psychol. Sci. 9, 397–401.

Andersson, S., Lundeberg, T., 1995. Acupuncture – from empiricism to science: functional background to acupuncture effects in pain and disease. Med. Hypotheses 45 (3), 271–281.

Andersson, U., Tracey, K.J., 2012. A new approach to rheumatoid arthritis: treating inflammation with computerized nerve stimulation. Cerebrum 3.

Anon, 1823. Acupuncturation. Lancet 200–201.

Baldry, P.E., 1993. Acupuncture, Trigger Points and Musculoskeletal Pain, second ed. Churchill Livingstone, Edinburgh. [use the 2005 edition only].

Baldry, P., 2005a. The integration of acupuncture within medicine in the UK – the British Medical Acupuncture Society's 25th anniversary. Acupuncture in Medicine 23 (1), 2–12.

Baldry, P.E., 2005b. Acupuncture, Trigger Points and Musculoskeletal Pain, third ed. Elsevier, Edinburgh.

Bally, M., Dendukuri, N., Rich, B., et al., 2017. Risk of acute myocardial infarction with NSAIDs in real world use: bayesian meta-analysis of individual patient data. BMJ 357, j1909.

Basser, S., 1999. Acupuncture: a history. Scientific Review of Alternative Medicine 3 (1), 34–41.

Berkovitz, S., Cummings, M., Perrin, C., Ito, R., 2008. High volume acupuncture clinic (HVAC) for chronic knee pain - audit of a possible model for delivery of acupuncture in the National Health Service. Acupunct. Med. 26, 46–50.

Birch, S., Kaptchuk, T., 1999. History, nature and current practice of acupuncture: an East Asian perspective. In: Ernst, E., White, A. (Eds.), Acupuncture: A Scientific Appraisal. Butterworth-Heinemann, Oxford, pp. 11–30.

Bivens, R.E., 2000. Acupuncture, Expertise and Cross-cultural Medicine. Palgrave, Manchester.

Brattberg, G., 1986. Acupuncture treatments: a traffic hazard? Am. J. Acupunct. 14, 265–267.

Brinkhaus, B., Ortiz, M., Witt, C.M., et al., 2013. Acupuncture in patients with seasonal allergic rhinitis. Ann. Intern. Med. 158, 225.

Brinkhaus, B., Witt, C.M., Jena, S., et al., 2008. Acupuncture in patients with allergic rhinitis: a pragmatic randomized trial. Ann. Allergy Asthma Immunol. 101 (5), 535–543.

Brumbaugh, A.G., 1993. Acupuncture: new perspectives in chemical dependency treatment. J. Subst. Abuse Treat. 10, 35–43.

Buckner, R.L., Andrews-Hanna, J.R., Schacter, D.L., 2008. The brain's default network: anatomy, function, and relevance to disease. Ann. N. Y. Acad. Sci. 1124, 1–38.

Campbell, A., 2001. Acupuncture in Practice: Beyond Points and Meridians. Butterworth-Heinemann, Oxford.

Cao, H., Li, X., Han, M., Liu, J., 2013. Acupoint stimulation for fibromyalgia: a systematic review of randomized controlled trials. Evidence-Based Complement Altern. Med 2013, 1–15.

Carr, D., 2015a. Somatosensory stimulation and assisted reproduction. Acupunct. Med. 33, 2–6.

Carr, D.J., 2015b. The safety of obstetric acupuncture: forbidden points revisited. Acupunct. Med. 33, 413–419.

Ceccherelli, F., Bordin, M., Gagliardi, G., et al., 2001. Comparison between superficial and deep acupuncture in the treatment of the shoulder's myofascial pain: a randomized and controlled study. Acupunct. Electrother Res. 26 (4), 229–238.

Ceccherelli, F., Gagliardi, G., Visentin, R., Giron, G., 1998. Effects of deep vs. superficial stimulation of acupuncture on capsaicin- induced edema. A blind controlled study in rats. Acupunct. Electrother Res. 23 (2), 125–134.

Chae, Y., Chang, D.S., Lee, S.H., et al., 2013. Inserting needles into the body: a meta-analysis of brain activity associated with acupuncture needle stimulation. J. Pain 14, 215–222.

Chang, B.H., Sommers, E., Herz, L., 2010. Acupuncture and the relaxation response for substance use disorder recovery. J. Subst. Use 15, 390–401.

Chang, H., Kwon, Y.D., Yoon, S.S., 2011. Use of acupuncture therapy as a supplement to conventional medical treatments for acute ischaemic stroke patients in an academic medical centre in Korea. Complement. Ther. Med. 19, 256–263.

Chapman, C.R., Chen, A.C., Bonica, J.J., 1977. Effects of intrasegmental electrical acupuncture on dental pain: evaluation by threshold estimation and sensory decision theory. Pain 3 (3), 213–227.

Chen, Y., 1997. Silk scrolls: earliest literature of meridian doctrine in ancient China. Acupunct. Electrother Res. 22, 175–189.

Cheng, L., Li, P., Tjen-A-Looi, S.C., Longhurst, J.C., 2015. What do we understand from clinical and mechanistic studies on acupuncture treatment for hypertension? Chin. Med. 10, 36.

Chiang, C.Y., Chang, C.T., Chu, H.L., et al., 1973. Peripheral afferent pathway for acupuncture analgesia. Sci. Sin. 16, 210.

Clement-Jones, V., McLoughlin, L., Tomlin, S., et al., 1980. Increased beta-endorphin but not met-enkephalin levels in human cerebrospinal fluid after acupuncture for recurrent pain. Lancet 316, 945–947.

Corbett, M.S., Rice, S.J.C., Madurasinghe, V., et al., 2013. Acupuncture and other physical treatments for the relief of pain due to osteoarthritis of the knee: network meta-analysis. Osteoarthr. Cartil. 21, 1290–1298.

Coyle, M., Smith, C., 2005. A survey comparing TCM diagnosis, health status and medical diagnosis in women undergoing assisted reproduction. Acupunct. Med. 23 (2), 62–69.

Cummings, M., 2009. Modellvorhaben Akupunktur - a summary of the ART, ARC and GERAC trials. Acupunct. Med. 27, 26–30.

Cummings, M., 2011. Safety aspects of electroacupuncture. Acupunct. Med. 29, 83–85.

Cummings, T.M., 1996. A computerised audit of acupuncture in two populations: civilian and forces. Acupunct. Med. 14, 37–39.

De Stefano, R., Selvi, E., Villanova, M., et al., 2000. Image analysis quantification of substance P immunoreactivity in the trapezius muscle of patients with fibromyalgia and myofascial pain syndrome. J. Rheumatol. 27 (12), 2906–2910.

Dhond, R.P., Yeh, C., Park, K., et al., 2008. Acupuncture modulates resting state connectivity in default and sensorimotor brain networks. Pain 136, 407–418.

Dodin, S., Blanchet, C., Marc, I., et al., 2013. Acupuncture for menopausal hot flushes. in: Dodin, S. (Ed.), Cochrane Database Syst. Rev. John Wiley & Sons, Ltd, Chichester, UK, CD007410.

Dorfer, L., Moser, M., Bahr, F., et al., 1999. A medical report from the stone age? Lancet 354, 1023–1025.

Dorfer, L., Moser, M., Spindler, K., et al., 1998. 5200-year-old acupuncture in Central Europe? [letter]. Science 282, 242–243.

Dyrehag, L.E., Widerstroem-Noga, E.G., Carlsson, S.G., et al., 1997. Effects of repeated sensory stimulation sessions (electro-acupuncture) on skin temperature in chronic pain patients. Scand. J. Rehabil. Med. 29, 243–250.

Ee, C.C., Manheimer, E., Pirotta, M.V., White, A.R., 2008. Acupuncture for pelvic and back pain in pregnancy: a systematic review. Am. J. Obstet. Gynecol. 198, 254–259.

Elden, H., Ladfors, L., Olsen, M.F., et al., 2005. Effects of acupuncture and stabilising exercises as adjunct to standard treatment in pregnant women with pelvic girdle pain: randomised single blind controlled trial. Br. Med. J. 330 (7494), 761–766.

Ernst, G., Strzyz, H., Hagmeister, H., 2003. Incidence of adverse effects during acupuncture therapy – a multicentre survey. Complement. Ther. Med. 11 (2), 93–97.

Fais, R.S., Reis, G.M., Rossaneis, A.C., et al., 2012. Amitriptyline converts non-responders into responders to low-frequency electroacupuncture-induced analgesia in rats. Life Sci. 91, 14–19.

Fang, J., Jin, Z., Wang, Y., et al., 2009. The salient characteristics of the central effects of acupuncture needling: limbic-paralimbic-neocortical network modulation. Hum. Brain Mapp. 30, 1196–1206.

Feng, S., Han, M., Fan, Y., et al., 2015. Acupuncture for the treatment of allergic rhinitis: A systematic review and meta-analysis. Am. J. Rhinol. Allergy 29, 57–62.

Filshie, J., 2001. Safety aspects of acupuncture in palliative care. Acupunct. Med. 19 (2), 117–122.

Filshie, J., Bolton, T., Browne, D., et al., 2005. Acupuncture and self acupuncture for long-term treatment of vasomotor symptoms in cancer patients – audit and treatment algorithm. Acupunct. Med. 23 (4), 171–180.

Filshie, J., Hester, J., 2006. Guidelines for providing acupuncture treatment for cancer patients – a peer-reviewed sample policy document. Acupunct. Med. 24 (4), 172–182.

Filshie, J., White, A., Cummings, M. (Eds.), 2016. Medical Acupuncture: A Western Scientific Approach, second ed. Elsevier, Edinburgh.

Fink, M., Wolkenstein, E., Karst, M., et al., 2002. Acupuncture in chronic epicondylitis: a randomized controlled trial. Rheumatology (Oxford) 41 (2), 205–209.

Foster, N.E., Bishop, A., Bartlam, B., et al., 2016. Evaluating acupuncture and standard care for pregnant women with Back pain (EASE Back): a feasibility study and pilot randomised trial. Health Technol Assess (Rockv) 20, 1–236.

Garcia, M.K., McQuade, J., Haddad, R., et al., 2013. Systematic review of acupuncture in cancer care: a synthesis of the evidence. J. Clin. Oncol. 31, 952–960.

Gerwin, R.D., Shannon, S., Hong, C.Z., et al., 1997. Interrater reliability in myofascial trigger point examination. Pain 69 (1–2), 65–73.

Goldman, N., Chandler-Militello, D., Langevin, H.M., et al., 2013. Purine receptor mediated actin cytoskeleton remodeling of human fibroblasts. Cell Calcium 53, 297–301.

Goldman, N., Chen, M., Fujita, T., et al., 2010. Adenosine A1 receptors mediate local anti-nociceptive effects of acupuncture. Nat. Neurosci. 13, 883–888.

Greenlee, H., DuPont-Reyes, M.J., Balneaves, L.G., et al., 2017. Clinical practice guidelines on the evidence-based use of integrative therapies during and after breast cancer treatment. CA Cancer J. Clin.

Greville-Harris, M., Hughes, J., Lewith, G., et al., 2016. Assessing knowledge about acupuncture: A survey of people with back pain in the UK. Complement. Ther. Med. 29, 164–168.

Gunn, C.C., 1996. The Gunn Approach to the Treatment of Chronic Pain. Churchill Livingstone, London.

Haker, E., Lundeberg, T., 1990. Acupuncture treatment in epicondylalgia: a comparative study of two acupuncture techniques. Clin. J. Pain 6, 221–226.

Han, J.S., 2004. Acupuncture and endorphins. Neurosci. Lett. 361 (1–3), 258–261.

Han, J., Cui, C., Wu, L., 2011. Acupuncture-related techniques for the treatment of opiate addiction: a case of translational medicine. Front Med. 5, 141–150.

Han, J., Terenius, L., 1982. Neurochemical basis of acupuncture analgesia. Annu. Rev. Pharmacol. Toxicol. 22, 193–220.

Harris, R.E., Zubieta, J.K., Scott, D.J., et al., 2009. Traditional Chinese acupuncture and placebo (sham) acupuncture are differentiated by their effects on mu-opioid receptors (MORs). Neuroimage 47, 1077–1085.

Helms, J.M., 1998. An overview of medical acupuncture. Altern. Ther. Health Med. 4 (3), 35–45.

Heo, I., Shin, B.C., Kim, Y.D., et al., 2013. Acupuncture for spinal cord injury and its complications: a systematic review and meta-analysis of randomized controlled trials. Evid. Based Complement. Alternat. Med. 2013, 364216.

Hernandez-Diaz, S., Rodriguez, L.A., 2000. Association between nonsteroidal anti-inflammatory drugs and upper gastrointestinal tract bleeding/perforation: an overview of epidemiologic studies published in the 1990s. Arch. Intern. Med. 160 (14), 2093–2099.

Hoffman, P., 2001. Skin disinfection and acupuncture. Acupunct. Med. 19 (2), 112–116.

Hong, C.Z., 2000. Myofascial trigger points: pathophysiology and correlation with acupuncture points. Acupunct. Med. 18 (1), 41–47.

Hong, C.Z., Kuan, T.S., Chen, J.T., et al., 1997. Referred pain elicited by palpation and by needling of myofascial trigger points: a comparison. Arch. Phys. Med. Rehabil. 78 (9), 957–960.

Hopton, A.K., Curnoe, S., Kanaan, M., Macpherson, H., 2012. Acupuncture in practice: mapping the providers, the patients and the settings in a national cross-sectional survey. BMJ Open 2, e000456.

Huang, W., Pach, D., Napadow, V., et al., 2012. Characterizing acupuncture stimuli using brain imaging with FMRI–a systematic review and meta-analysis of the literature. PLoS ONE 7, e32960.

Hubbard, D.R., Berkoff, G.M., 1993. Myofascial trigger points show EMG activity. Spine 18, 1803–1807.

Hughes, J., Smith, T.W., Kosterlitz, H.W., et al., 1975. Identification of two related pentapeptides from the brain with potent opiate agonist activity. Nature 258 (5536), 577–580.

Hui, K.K., Liu, J., Makris, N., et al., 2000. Acupuncture modulates the limbic system and subcortical gray structures of the human brain: evidence from fMRI studies in normal subjects. Hum. Brain Mapp. 9 (1), 13–25.

Hui, K.K.S., Liu, J., Marina, O., et al., 2005. The integrated response of the human cerebro-cerebellar and limbic systems to acupuncture stimulation at ST 36 as evidenced by fMRI. Neuroimage 27 (3), 479–496.

Kaplan, G., 1997. A brief history of acupuncture's journey to the West. J. Altern. Complement. Med. 3, S5S10.

Kaptchuk, T., 1983. Chinese Medicine: The Web That has no Weaver. Rider, London.

Kelleher, C.J., Filshie, J., Burton, G., et al., 1994. Acupuncture and the treatment of irritative bladder symptoms. Acupunct. Med. 12 (1), 9–12.

Kellgren, J.H., 1938. Observations on referred pain arising from muscle. Clin. Sci. 3, 175–190.

Kendall, D.E., 2002. Dao of Chinese Medicine: Understanding an Ancient Healing Art. Oxford University Press, New York.

Kim, S.Y., Lee, H., Chae, Y., Park, H.J., 2012. A systematic review of cost-effectiveness analyses alongside randomised controlled trials of acupuncture. Acupunct. Med. 30, 273–285.

Kong, J., Kaptchuk, T.J., Polich, G., et al., 2009. Expectancy and treatment interactions: a dissociation between acupuncture analgesia and expectancy evoked placebo analgesia. Neuroimage 45, 940–949.

Lagrue, G., Poupy, J.L., Grillot, A., et al., 1977. Acupuncture anti-tabagique. La Nouvelle Presse Médicale 9, 966.

Langevin, H.M., Churchill, D.L., Fox, J.R., et al., 2001. Biomechanical response to acupuncture needling in humans. J. Appl. Physiol. 91, 2471–2478.

Langevin, H.M., Storch, K.N., Cipolla, M.J., et al., 2006. Fibroblast spreading induced by connective tissue stretch involves intracellular redistribution of alpha- and beta-actin. Histochem. Cell Biol. 125, 487–495.

Lawson-Wood, D., Lawson-Wood, J., 1973. The Five Elements of Acupuncture and Chinese Massage. Health Science Press, Holsworthy, Devon.

Lee, A., Chan, S.K., Fan, L.T., 2015. Stimulation of the wrist acupuncture point PC6 for preventing postoperative nausea and vomiting. in: Lee, A. (Ed.), Cochrane Database Syst. Rev. John Wiley & Sons, Ltd, Chichester, UK, CD003281.

Lewith, G.T., Kenyon, J.N., Broomfield, J., et al., 2001. Is electrodermal testing as effective as skin prick tests for diagnosing allergies? A double blind, randomised block design study. Br. Med. J. 322 (7279), 131–134.

Li, C., Ji, B.U., Kim, Y., et al., 2016. Electroacupuncture Enhances the Antiallodynic and Antihyperalgesic Effects of Milnacipran in Neuropathic Rats. Anesth. Analg. 122, 1654–1662.

Li, J., Zhang, J.H., Yi, T., et al., 2014. Acupuncture treatment of chronic low back pain reverses an abnormal brain default mode network in correlation with clinical pain relief. Acupunct. Med. 32, 102–108.

Li, P., Tjen-A-Looi, S.C., Cheng, L., et al., 2015. Long-lasting reduction of blood pressure by electroacupuncture in patients with hypertension: RCT. Med. Acupunct. 27, 253–266.

Liddle, S.D., Pennick, V., 2015. Interventions for preventing and treating low-back and pelvic pain during pregnancy. in: Liddle, S.D. (Ed.), Cochrane Database Syst. Rev. John Wiley & Sons, Ltd, Chichester, UK, CD001139.

Lin, X., Huang, K., Zhu, G., et al., 2016a. The effects of acupuncture on chronic knee pain due to osteoarthritis. J. Bone Jt. Surg. 98, 1578–1585.

Lin, Y.J., Kung, Y.Y., Kuo, W.J., et al., 2016b. Effect of acupuncture "dose" on modulation of the default mode network of the brain. Acupunct. Med. 34, 425–432.

Lindall, S., 1999. Is acupuncture for pain relief in general practice cost-effective? Acupunct. Med. 17 (2), 97–100.

Linde, K., Allais, G., Brinkhaus, B., et al., 2016a. Acupuncture for the prevention of episodic migraine. in: Linde, K. (Ed.), Cochrane Database Syst. Rev. John Wiley & Sons, Ltd, Chichester, UK, CD001218.

Linde, K., Allais, G., Brinkhaus, B., et al., 2016b. Acupuncture for the prevention of tension-type headache. in: Linde, K. (Ed.), Cochrane Database Syst. Rev. John Wiley & Sons, Ltd, Chichester, UK, CD007587.

Linde, K., Streng, A., Hoppe, A., et al., 2006. The programme for the evaluation of patient care with acupuncture (PEP-Ac) – a project sponsored by ten German social health insurance funds. Acupunct. Med. 24 (Suppl.), 25–32.

Long, X., Huang, W., Napadow, V., et al., 2016. Sustained effects of acupuncture stimulation investigated with centrality mapping analysis. Front. Hum. Neurosci. 10, 510.

Lu, G.D., Needham, J., 1980. Celestial Lancets: a History and Rationale of Acupuncture and Moxa. Cambridge University Press, Cambridge.

Lund, I., Lundeberg, T., 2006. Are minimal, superficial or sham acupuncture procedures acceptable as inert placebo controls? Acupunct. Med. 24 (1), 13–15.

Lundeberg, T., 1999. Effects of sensory stimulation (acupuncture) on circulatory and immune systems. In: Ernst, E., White, A. (Eds.), Acupuncture: A Scientific Appraisal. Butterworth-Heinemann, Oxford.

Lundeberg, T., Bondesson, L., Thomas, M., 1987. Effect of acupuncture on experimentally induced itch. Br. J. Dermatol. 117 (6), 771–777.

Lundeberg, T., Eriksson, S., Lundeberg, S., Thomas, M., 1989. Acupuncture and sensory thresholds. Am. J. Chin. Med. 17 (3–4), 99–110.

Lundeberg, T., Lund, I., Näslund, J.M.T., 2009. The Emperor's sham - wrong assumption that sham needling is sham. Acupunct. Med. 26 (4), 239–242.

Ma, K.W., 1992. The roots and development of Chinese acupuncture: from prehistory to early 20th century. Acupunct. Med. 10 (Suppl.), 92–99.

MacDonald, A.J.R., 1982. Acupuncture: from Ancient Art to Modern Medicine, first ed. George Allen & Unwin, Boston.

Maciocia, G., 1989. The Foundations of Chinese Medicine. Churchill Livingstone, Edinburgh.

MacPherson, H., Thomas, K., 2005. Short term reactions to acupuncture – a cross-sectional survey of patient reports. Acupunct. Med. 23 (3), 112–120.

MacPherson, H., Thomas, K., Walters, S., et al., 2001. A prospective survey of adverse events and treatment reactions following 34,000 consultations with professional acupuncturists. Acupunct. Med. 19 (2), 93–102.

Mann, F., 1992. Reinventing Acupuncture. Butterworth Heinemann, Oxford.

Mayer, D.J., Price, D.D., Rafii, A., 1977. Antagonism of acupuncture analgesia in man by the narcotic antagonist naloxone. Brain Res. 121, 368–372.

Melchart, D., Thormaehlen, J., Hager, S., et al., 2003. Acupuncture versus placebo versus sumatriptan for early treatment of migraine attacks: a randomized controlled trial. J. Intern. Med. 253 (2), 181–188.

Melzack, R., Stillwell, D.M., Fox, E.J., 1977. Trigger points and acupuncture points for pain: correlations and implications. Pain 3, 3–23.

Melzack, R., Wall, P.D., 1965. Pain mechanisms: a new theory. Science 150 (699), 971–979.

Melzack, R., Wall, P.D., 1988. The Challenge of Pain. Penguin Books, London.

Mense, S., Simons, D.G., 1999. Muscle Pain: Understanding Its Nature, Diagnosis and Treatment. Lippincott Williams & Wilkins, Philadelphia.

Molsberger, A.F., Schneider, T., Gotthardt, H., Drabik, A., 2010. German Randomized Acupuncture Trial for chronic shoulder pain (GRASP) - a pragmatic, controlled, patient-blinded, multi-centre trial in an outpatient care environment. Pain 151, 146–154.

Myers, C.P., 1991. Acupuncture in general practice: effect on drug expenditure. Acupunct. Med. 9, 71–72.

Napadow, V., Kettner, N.W., Harris, R.E., 2016. Neuroimaging: a window into human brain mechanisms supporting acupuncture effects, in: Medical Acupuncture: A Western Scientific Approach, pp. 59–72.

Napadow, V., Kim, J., Clauw, D.J., Harris, R.E., 2012. Decreased intrinsic brain connectivity is associated with reduced clinical pain in fibromyalgia. Arthritis Rheum. 64, 2398–2403.

Nesheim, B.I., Kinge, R., 2006. Performance of acupuncture as labor analgesia in the clinical setting. Acta Obstet. Gynecol. Scand. 85 (4), 441–443.

Nguyen, V.T.T., McLaws, M.L., Dore, G.J., 2007. Highly endemic hepatitis B infection in rural Vietnam. J. Gastroenterol. Hepatol. 22, 2093–2100.

NIH Consensus Development Panel, 1998. NIH Consensus Conference. Acupuncture. JAMA 280 (17), 1518–1524.

Nogier, P.M.F., 1981. Handbook to Auriculotherapy. Maisonneuve, Moulin-les-Metz.

Oomman, S., Liu, D., Cummings, M., 2005. Acupuncture for acute postoperative pain relief in a patient with pregnancy-induced thrombocytopenia – a case report. Acupunct. Med. 23 (2), 83–85.

Osler, W., 1912. The Principles and Practice of Medicine, eighth ed. Appleton, New York.

Pariente, J., White, P., Frackowiak, R.S., et al., 2005. Expectancy and belief modulate the neuronal substrates of pain treated by acupuncture. Neuroimage 25 (4), 1161–1167.

Park, J., White, A.R., Lee, H., Ernst, E., 1999. Development of a new sham needle. Acupunct. Med. 17, 110–112.

Peuker, E., Cummings, M., 2003a. Anatomy for the acupuncturist – facts & fiction. 1: the head and neck region. Acupunct. Med. 21 (1–2), 2–8.

Peuker, E., Cummings, M., 2003b. Anatomy for the acupuncturist – facts & fiction. 2: the chest, abdomen, and back. Acupunct. Med. 21 (3), 72–79.

Peuker, E., Cummings, M., 2003c. Anatomy for the acupuncturist – facts & fiction. 3: upper & lower extremity. Acupunct. Med. 21 (4), 122–132.

Pham, D.D., Yoo, J.H., Tran, B.Q., Ta, T.T., 2013. Complementary and alternative medicine use among physicians in oriental medicine hospitals in Vietnam: A hospital-based survey. Evidence-Based Complement Altern. Med 2013, 1–9.

Pomeranz, B., 2001. Acupuncture analgesia – basic research. In: Stux, G., Hammerschlag, R. (Eds.), Clinical Acupuncture – Scientific Basis. Springer, Berlin.

Pomeranz, B., Chiu, D., 1976. Naloxone blockade of acupuncture analgesia: endorphin implicated. Life Sci. 19 (11), 1757–1762.

Pullman, M., 2016. Acupuncture for urogenital conditions. In: Medical Acupuncture: A Western Scientific Approach, second ed. Elsevier, Amsterdam, pp. 475–488.

Qin, Z., Wu, J., Zhou, J., Liu, Z., 2016. Systematic review of acupuncture for chronic prostatitis/chronic pelvic pain syndrome. Medicine (Baltimore) 95, e3095.

Ratcliffe, J., Thomas, K.J., MacPherson, H., et al., 2006. A randomised controlled trial of acupuncture care for persistent low back pain: cost effectiveness analysis. Br. Med. J. 333 (7569), 626–628A.

Reinhold, T., Roll, S., Willich, S.N., et al., 2013. Cost-effectiveness for acupuncture in seasonal allergic rhinitis: economic results of the ACUSAR trial. Ann. Allergy Asthma Immunol. 111, 56–63.

Reinhold, T., Witt, C.M., Jena, S., et al., 2008. Quality of life and cost-effectiveness of acupuncture treatment in patients with osteoarthritis pain. Eur. J. Heal Econ 9, 209–219.

Research Group of Acupuncture Anaesthesia, 1974. The role of some neurotransmitters of brain in finger-acupuncture analgesia. Sci. Sin. 17, 112–130.

Reston, J., 1971. Now about my operation in Peking. New York Times 1, 6.

Ross, J., 2001. An audit of the impact of introducing microacupuncture into primary care. Acupunct. Med. 19 (1), 43–45.

Ross, J., White, A., Ernst, E., 1999. Western, minimal acupuncture for neck pain: a cohort study. Acupunct. Med. 17 (1), 5–8.

Sandberg, M., Lundeberg, T., Lindberg, L.G., et al., 2003. Effects of acupuncture on skin and muscle blood flow in healthy subjects. Eur. J. Appl. Physiol. 90 (1–2), 114–119.

Sato, A., Sato, Y., Suzuki, A., Uchida, S., 1993. Neural mechanisms of the reflex inhibition and excitation of gastric motility elicited by acupuncture-like stimulation in anesthetized rats. Neurosci. Res. 18 (1), 53–62.

Schnorrenberger, C.C., 2003. Chen-Chiu: the Original Acupuncture, a New Healing Paradigm. Wisdom Publications, Somerville, MA.

Sciotti, V.M., Mittak, V.L., DiMarco, L., et al., 2001. Clinical precision of myofascial trigger point location in the trapezius muscle. Pain 93 (3), 259–266.

Shah, J.P., Phillips, T.M., Danoff, J.V., et al., 2005. An in vivo microanalytical technique for measuring the local biochemical milieu of human skeletal muscle. J. Appl. Physiol. 99 (5), 1977–1984.

Shen, J., Wenger, N., Glaspy, J., et al., 2000. Electroacupuncture for control of myeloablative chemotherapy-induced emesis: A randomized controlled trial. J. Am. Med. Assoc. 284, 2755–2761.

Shin, N.Y., Lim, Y.J., Yang, C.H., Kim, C., 2017. Acupuncture for alcohol use disorder: a meta-analysis. Evidence-Based Complement Altern. Med 2017, 1–6.

Simons, D.G., Travell, J.G., Simons, L.S., 1999. Myofascial Pain and Dysfunction: the Trigger Point Manual, vol. 1, second ed. Upper half of body. Williams & Wilkins, Baltimore.

Skootsky, S.A., Jaeger, B., Oye, R.K., 1989. Prevalence of myofascial pain in general internal medicine practice. Western Journal of Medicine 151 (2), 157–160.

Smith, C.A., 2016. Acupuncture in obstetrics. In: Medical Acupuncture: A Western Scientific Approach. Elsevier, Amsterdam, pp. 552–565.

Smith, C.A., Armour, M., Zhu, X., et al., 2016. Acupuncture for dysmenorrhoea. Cochrane Database Syst. Rev. CD007854, in: Smith, C.A. (Ed.), John Wiley & Sons, Ltd, Chichester, UK.

Smith, C.A., Collins, C.T., Crowther, C.A., Levett, K.M., 2011. Acupuncture or acupressure for pain management in labour. Cochrane Database Syst. Rev. CD009232.

Sola, A.E., Rodenberger, M.L., Gettys, B.B., 1955. Incidence of hypersensitive areas in posterior shoulder muscles. Am. J. Phys. Med. 3, 585–590.

Soulié de Morant, G., 1957. L'Acuponcture Chinoise. J. Lafitte, Paris.

Spaeth, R.B., Camhi, S., Hashmi, J.A., et al., 2013. A longitudinal study of the reliability of acupuncture deqi sensations in knee osteoarthritis. Evidence-Based Complement Altern. Med. 2013, 1–12.

Stener-Victorin, E., 2016. Acupuncture in gynaecology and infertility. In: Medical Acupuncture: A Western Scientific Approach. Elsevier, Amsterdam.

Stener-Victorin, E., Humaidan, P., 2006. Use of acupuncture in female infertility and a summary of recent acupuncture studies related to embryo transfer. Acupunct. Med. 24 (4), 157–163.

Stener-Victorin, E., Jedel, E., Janson, P.O., Sverrisdottir, Y.B., 2009. Low-frequency electroacupuncture and physical exercise decrease high muscle sympathetic nerve activity in polycystic ovary syndrome. Am. J. Physiol. Regul. Integr. Comp. Physiol. 297, R387–R395.

Stener-Victorin, E., Kobayashi, R., Kurosawa, M., 2003. Ovarian blood flow responses to electro-acupuncture stimulation at different frequencies and intensities in anaesthetized rats. Auton. Neurosci. 108, 50–56.

Stener-Victorin, E., Kobayashi, R., Watanabe, O., et al., 2004. Effect of electro-acupuncture stimulation of different frequencies and intensities on ovarian blood flow in anaesthetized rats with steroid-induced polycystic ovaries. Reprod. Biol. Endocrinol. 2, 16.

Streitberger, K., Kleinhenz, J., 1998. Introducing a placebo needle into acupuncture research. Lancet 352, 364–365.

Stuyt, E.B., 2014. Ear acupuncture for co-occurring substance abuse and borderline personality disorder: an aid to encourage treatment retention and tobacco cessation. Acupunct. Med. 32 (4), 318–324.

Takakura, N., Takayama, M., Kawase, A., Yajima, H., 2011. Double blinding with a new placebo needle: a validation study on participant blinding. Acupunct. Med. 29 (3), 203–207.

Tang, H., Fan, H., Chen, J., et al., 2015. Acupuncture for lateral epicondylitis: a systematic review. Evidence-Based Complement Altern. Med 2015, 1–13.

The Academy of Traditional Chinese Medicine, 1975. An Outline of Chinese Acupuncture. Foreign Languages Press, Peking.

Thomas, K.J., MacPherson, H., Ratcliffe, J., et al., 2005. Longer term clinical and economic benefits of offering acupuncture care to patients with chronic low back pain. Health Technol. Assess. Rep. 9 (32), 1–126.

Thomas, K.J., Nicholl, J.P., Coleman, P., 2001. Use and expenditure on complementary medicine in England: a population based survey. Complement Therapies in Medicine 9 (1), 2–11.

Thomas, M., Eriksson, S.V., Lundeberg, T., 1991. A comparative study of diazepam and acupuncture in patients with osteoarthritis. Am. J. Chin. Med. 19, 95–100.

Thomas, M., Lundeberg, T., Björk, G., et al., 1995. Pain and discomfort in primary dysmenorrhoea is reduced by preemptive acupuncture or low frequency TENS. European Journal of Physical and Medical Rehabilitation 5 (3), 71–76.

Torres-Rosas, R., Yehia, G., Peña, G., et al., 2014. Dopamine mediates vagal modulation of the immune system by electroacupuncture. Nat. Med. 20, 291–295.

Tough, E.A., White, A.R., Cummings, T.M., et al., 2009. Acupuncture and dry needling in the management of myofascial trigger point pain: a systematic review and meta-analysis of randomised controlled trials. Eur. J. Pain 13, 3–10.

Tough, E.A., White, A.R., Richards, S., et al., 2007. Variability of criteria used to diagnose myofascial trigger point pain syndrome – evidence from a review of the literature. Clin. J. Pain 23 (3), 278–286.

Tracey, K.J., 2002. The inflammatory reflex. Nature 420, 853–859.

Travell, J.G., Simons, D.G., 1983. Myofascial Pain and Dysfunction: The Trigger Point Manual, first ed. Williams & Wilkins, Baltimore.

Travell, J.G., Simons, D.G., 1992. Myofascial Pain and Dysfunction: The Trigger Point Manual, vol. 2, first ed. The Lower Extremities. Williams & Wilkins, Baltimore.

Ulett, G., 1992. Beyond Yin and Yang: How Acupuncture Really Works. Warren H Green, St. Louis.

Ulett, G.A., Han, S.P., 2002. The Biology of Acupuncture. Warren H Green, St. Louis.

Uvnas-Moberg, K., Bruzelius, G., Alster, P., et al., 1993. The antinociceptive effect of non-noxious sensory stimulation is mediated partly through oxytocinergic mechanisms. Acta Physiol. Scand. 149, 199–204.

Van den Heuvel, E., Goossens, M., Vanderhaegen, H., et al., 2015. Effect of acustimulation on nausea and vomiting and on hyperemesis in pregnancy: a systematic review of Western and Chinese literature. BMC Complement. Altern. Med. 16, 13.

Vas, J., Ortega, C., Olmo, V., et al., 2008. Single-point acupuncture and physiotherapy for the treatment of painful shoulder: a multicentre randomized controlled trial. Rheumatology 47, 887–993.

Veith, I., 1949. The Yellow Emperor's Classic of Internal Medicine. University of California Press, Berkeley.

Vickers, A.J., Cronin, A.M., Maschino, A.C., et al., 2012. Acupuncture for Chronic Pain: Individual Patient Data Meta-analysis. Arch. Intern. Med. 172, 1444–1453.

Vickers, A.J., Vertosick, E.A., Lewith, G., et al., 2017. Acupuncture for Chronic Pain: Update of an Individual Patient Data Meta-Analysis. J. Pain doi:10.1016/j.jpain.2017.11.005. (Published Online First: 30 November 2017.)

Vida, G., Peña, G., Deitch, E.A., Ulloa, L., 2011. α7-cholinergic receptor mediates vagal induction of splenic norepinephrine. J. Immunol. 186, 4340–4346.

Vincent, C., 2001. The safety of acupuncture. Br. Med. J. 323 (7311), 467–468.

Vincent, C.A., Richardson, P.H., Black, J.J., et al., 1989. The significance of needle placement site in acupuncture. J. Psychosom. Res. 33, 489–496.

Vohra, S., Adams, D., Yasui, Y., et al., 2011. The safety of pediatric acupuncture: a systematic review. Pediatrics 128, e1575–e1587.

Walsh, B., 2001. Control of infection in acupuncture. Acupunct. Med. 19 (2), 109–111.

Wang, K., Yao, S., Xian, Y., et al., 1985. A study of the receptive field of acupoints and the relationship between the characteristics of needling sensation and groups of afferent fibres. Sci. Sin. 28, 963.

Wang, R., Li, X., Zhou, S., et al., 2017. Manual acupuncture for myofascial pain syndrome: a systematic review and meta-analysis. Acupunct. Med. 35 (4), 241–250.

Wardle, J.L., Sibbritt, D., Adams, J., 2013. Acupuncture referrals in rural primary healthcare: a survey of general practitioners in rural and regional New South Wales, Australia. Acupunct. Med. 31, 375–382.

Wedenberg, K., Moen, B., Norling, A., 2000. A prospective randomized study comparing acupuncture with physiotherapy for low-back and pelvic pain in pregnancy. Acta Obstet. Gynecol. Scand. 79 (5), 331–335.

Wen, H.L., Cheung, S.Y.C., 1973. Treatment of drug addiction by acupuncture and electrical stimulation. Asian Med. J. 9, 138–141.

Wheway, J., Agbabiaka, T.B., Ernst, E., 2012. Patient safety incidents from acupuncture treatments: a review of reports to the National Patient Safety Agency. Int. J. Risk Saf. Med. 24, 163–169.

White, A., 2004. A cumulative review of the range and incidence of significant adverse events associated with acupuncture. Acupunct. Med. 22 (3), 122–133.

White, A., 2006. The safety of acupuncture – evidence from the UK. Acupunct. Med. 24 (Suppl.), S53S57.

White, A., 2013. Trials of acupuncture for drug dependence: a recommendation for hypotheses based on the literature. Acupunct. Med. 31, 297–304.

White, A., Foster, N.E., Cummings, M., et al., 2007. Acupuncture treatment for chronic knee pain: a systematic review. Rheumatology (Oxford) 46 (3), 384–390.

White, A., Hayhoe, S., Hart, A., et al., 2001. Survey of adverse events following acupuncture (SAFA): a prospective study of 32,000 consultations. Acupunct. Med. 19 (2), 84–92.

White, A., Richardson, M., Richmond, P., et al., 2012. Group acupuncture for knee pain: evaluation of a cost-saving initiative in the health service. Acupunct. Med. 30, 170–175.

White, A.R., Rampes, H., Liu, J.P., et al., 2014. Acupuncture and related interventions for smoking cessation. Cochrane Database Syst. Rev. (1), CD000009.

Willich, S.N., Reinhold, T., Selim, D., et al., 2006. Cost-effectiveness of acupuncture treatment in patients with chronic neck pain. Pain 125, 107–113.

Witt, C.M., Brinkhaus, B., Reinhold, T., et al., 2006a. Efficacy, effectiveness, safety and costs of acupuncture for chronic pain – results of a large research initiative. Acupunct. Med. 24 (Suppl.), S33S39.

Witt, C.M., Jena, S., Brinkhaus, B., et al., 2006b. Acupuncture in patients with osteoarthritis of the knee or hip: a randomized, controlled trial with an additional nonrandomized arm. Arthritis Rheum. 54 (11), 3485–3493.

Witt, C.M., Jena, S., Selim, D., et al., 2006c. Pragmatic randomized trial evaluating the clinical and economic effectiveness of acupuncture for chronic low back pain. Am. J. Epidemiol. 164 (5), 487–496.

Witt, C.M., Reinhold, T., Jena, S., et al., 2008a. Cost-effectiveness of acupuncture treatment in patients with headache. Cephalalgia 28, 334–345.

Witt, C.M., Reinhold, T., Brinkhaus, B., et al., 2008b. Acupuncture in patients with dysmenorrhea: a randomized study on clinical effectiveness and cost-effectiveness in usual care. Am. J. Obstet. Gynecol. 198, 166.e1–166.e8.

Witt, C.M., Pach, D., Brinkhaus, B., et al., 2009. Safety of acupuncture: results of a prospective observational study with 229,230 patients and introduction of a medical information and consent form. Forsch. Komplementarmed. 16, 91–97.

Wolfe, F., Smythe, H.A., Yunus, M.B., et al., 1990. The American College of Rheumatology 1990 Criteria for the classification of fibromyalgia. Report of the Multicenter Criteria Committee. Arthritis Rheum. 33 (2), 160–172.

Wonderling, D., Vickers, A.J., Grieve, R., et al., 2004. Cost effectiveness analysis of a randomised trial of acupuncture for chronic headache in primary care. Br. Med. J. 328 (7442), 747–749.

Woolf, C.J., 1996. Windup and central sensitization are not equivalent. Pain 66 (2–3), 105–108.

Woollam, C.H.M., Jackson, A.O., 1998. Acupuncture in the management of chronic pain. Anaesthesia 53 (6), 593–595.

Wu, M.T., Sheen, J.M., Chuang, K.H., et al., 2002. Neuronal specificity of acupuncture response: a fMRI study with electroacupuncture. Neuroimage 16 (4), 1028–1037.

Wyon, Y., Lindgren, R., Lundeberg, T., et al., 1995. Effects of acupuncture on climacteric vasomotor symptoms, quality of life, and urinary excretion of neuropeptides among postmenopausal women. Menopause 2, 3–12.

Xie, Y.M., Xu, S., Zhang, C.S., Xue, C.C., 2014. Examination of surface conditions and other physical properties of commonly used stainless steel acupuncture needles. Acupunct. Med. 32, 146–154.

Xu, S., Wang, L., Cooper, E., et al., 2013. Adverse events of acupuncture: a systematic review of case reports. Evidence-based Complement Altern. Med 2013, 581203.

Yamashita, H., Tsukayama, H., Tanno, Y., et al., 1999. Adverse events in acupuncture and moxibustion treatment: a six-year survey at a national clinic in Japan. J. Altern. Complement. Med. 5 (3), 229–236.

Yang, H.P., Wang, L., Han, L., Wang, S.C., 2013. Nonsocial Functions of Hypothalamic Oxytocin. ISRN Neurosci 2013, 1–13.

Yang, J., Yang, Y., Chen, J.M., et al., 2007. Effect of oxytocin on acupuncture analgesia in the rat. Neuropeptides 41, 285–292.

Yoon, S.S., Kwon, Y.K., Kim, M.R., et al., 2004. Acupuncture-mediated inhibition of ethanol-induced dopamine release in the rat nucleus accumbens through the GABA-B receptor. Neurosci. Lett. 369 (3), 234–238.

Yuan, Q., Guo, T., Liu, L., et al., 2015. Traditional Chinese medicine for neck pain and low back pain: a systematic review and meta-analysis. PLoS ONE 10, e0117146.

Yue, J., Zhang, Q., Sun, Z., et al., 2013. A case of electroacupuncture therapy for pressure ulcer. Acupunct. Med. 31, 450–451.

Zhao, Z.Q., 2008. Neural mechanism underlying acupuncture analgesia. Prog. Neurobiol. 85, 355–375.

Page numbers followed by "*f*" indicate figures, "*t*" indicate tables, and "*b*" indicate boxes.